JULIA BUCKROYD trained as a counsellor at Birkbeck College at the University of London and then as a psychotherapist with the Guild of Psychotherapists. For five years she was the student counsellor at the London Contemporary Dance School and then a therapist in private practice. She is now also Principal Lecturer in Counselling at the University of Hertfordshire. She has a continuing particular interest in eating disorders and has developed innovative ways of working with groups of eating disordered people as well as with individuals. She also offers training and workshops to those with an interest in developing their competence in this field as counsellors or therapists.

She was educated first as an academic historian at St. Andrews University, McMaster University in Hamilton, Ontario, at Cambridge and then Oxford University. As her interests have changed and developed, she has written extensively on a wide range of subjects, from Scottish history, to dance, to bereavement and other aspects of counselling and therapy.

Eating Your Heart Out

Understanding and overcoming eating disorders

Julia Buckroyd

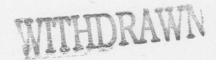

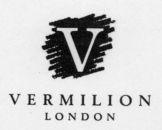

VERMILION
LONDON

First published in Great Britain in 1989 by Macdonald Optima.
Revised edition published by Optima in 1994.

1 3 5 7 9 10 8 6 4 2

This edition published in the United Kingdom in 1996 by Vermilion, an imprint of Ebury Press.

Random House UK Ltd
Random House
20 Vauxhall Bridge Road
London SW1V 2SA

Random House Australia (Pty) Ltd
20 Alfred Street
Milsons Point Sydney
New South Wales 2016 Australia

Random House New Zealand Limited
18 Poland Road, Glanfield
Aukland 10 New Zealand

Random House South Africa (Pty) Limited
PO Box 2263 Rosebank 2121 South Africa

Random House UK Limited Reg. No. 954009

A CIP catalogue record for this book is available from the British Library

ISBN 0 09 181502 9

Printed and bound in Great Britain by Mackays of Chatham, plc

Papers used by Vermilion are natural, recyclable products made from wood grown in sustainable forests.

Contents

For dearest B
without whom not

Preface

Ten years ago as an academic with pastoral responsibility for up to fifty women college students at any one time, I began to be aware of the prevalence of eating disorders among female students. My first conscious acknowledgement of this problem among the women whose welfare was my concern came when a worried landlady phoned to tell me that one of them seemed to be surviving on about 300 calories a day. It was the beginning of a long-term attempt to understand problems with food, eating, weight and size. That process continued through my decision to leave the academic world and retrain as a counsellor and has developed over the past five years in my work as student counsellor at London Contemporary Dance School as well as with the clients I see privately.

During this time I have had ample opportunity to reflect on my own eating behaviour and my own use of food. I have become aware of how, at particularly stressful times during my life, I have become what I should now describe as anorexic and lost significant amounts of weight. I have also been able to recognise what I now think of as many anorexic episodes when some disturbing event or experience has made me vow not to eat for the next day or few. I have also had to acknowledge that since my teens there have been times when I have binged and then vomited and many more times when I have just binged, especially late at night when I have not been able to sleep. I count myself happy that these ways of trying to deal with emotional pain have never taken over my life for all that long and have never been clinically diagnosed; the longest anorexic time lasted a little less than a year. However, I also know that I am still capable of eating nothing because my heart hurts or of eating more than I want for the same reason. I am glad that it is now some years since I have made myself sick. It has taken me a long time to feel kinder to myself and to be more accepting of my pain.

This book, therefore, is not written from the position of someone who is happy in the knowledge that she is not troubled by these difficult problems. I have some idea of how much anguish eating disorders can cause the sufferer. When I first began to read books on the subject in the late seventies I was very put off by the distant, lofty, superior and often punishing tone of much that was written by their usually male, often medical, authors. Anorexics were labelled sly and deceitful, bulimics disgusting, compulsive eaters greedy and untruthful. I found something voyeuristic in their descriptions of binges or bulimic episodes. Their concentration on medical diagnoses, physical symptoms and violent solutions – operations, administrations of drugs, forced feeding, behavioural conditioning programmes, aversion therapy – seemed to me then, and does now, unlikely to help women who are seriously disturbed to regain a sense of themselves and a respect and love for their own bodies. It is my experience that people with eating disorders are all too ready to insult and attack themselves both physically and verbally. Further attacks from those who want to help seem unlikely to be useful.

At the basis of any therapeutic endeavour there needs to develop an alliance, a trust, a co-operation, a mutual respect. We none of us want to have good done to us, at the expense of our dignity and our pride. I have tried to incorporate these ideals in these pages. You, the reader, are in the end responsible for yourself and your own behaviour. You may need some help, but you are the one who has to want it and to take it. Nobody can make you better against your will. This book invites you to take an active part in looking at your own behaviour and in considering how your own experiences are reflected in what is described.

Eating disorders are now the commonest symptom with which women in our society express their distress. The scale of the problem is enormous, especially at a sub-clinical level. Perhaps not all that many are so ill that they find their way to a doctor; that does not mean that they do not have a problem. When eating disorders were perceived as affecting only a small group within the population then it might have made sense (though I doubt it) to explain them by reference to one theory. The one that was most often suggested was that women with eating disorders had problems with growing up and especially with their sexuality. This may be true for some, but not for all. Most recently feminists have suggested that eating disorders are women's unconscious response to the social role in which society places them. I respect feminists' work enormously and think it is by far the most exciting and creative work done in recent years, but I still do not believe that all eating disorders can be understood by reference to this, or any, one theory.

What I have attempted here is to present a *range* of ways of understanding and thinking about the emotional meaning of eating disorders. It is your role to consider where you fit in. There may be more than one way of thinking about your difficulties. Perhaps none of what follows will match your situation exactly, but I hope you will get some clues about what is going on when you find yourself using your eating behaviour as a means of expressing your emotional pain.

The experience on which this book is written is very largely my work as a counsellor working with young women between the ages of 16 and 25. This group has been multi-racial, although predominantly white, and across a socio-economic spectrum from working class to upper middle class. It has included a few men, but only a few and all of them young; and a few older middle-class women, but only a few. I have not worked with people in their early teens. My experience, therefore, has the limitations imposed by the restrictions of the sample of the populations with whom I have worked.

The names and details of the case histories have been altered to make the people concerned unidentifiable, except perhaps to themselves. In some instances a number of similar stories have been put together and in others one story has been presented as several separate histories. This has been done to protect further the identity of those with whom I have worked, as well as to illustrate what I am saying. Some of the histories presented I have learned of from colleagues. Some of my clients have known that I was writing this book and have kindly offered me diaries, poems and other writing to use. I would like to thank them for their generosity. I would also like to record my respect for those sufferers from eating disorders who, with great courage, have shared their pain and distress. What I know about the subject I have learned largely from them.

I would also like to express my thanks to those without whom this book would not have been written: first of all to my colleagues at London Contemporary Dance School. My time in the school as student counsellor is made more enjoyable by their friendship and support. I am given space, time and opportunity to develop counselling work and attitudes within the school and although my ideas and activities do not always meet with their agreement, they are respected. I owe a particular debt of gratitude to the Principal of the school, Richard Ralph, and to the body-conditioning teacher, Sonia Noonan.

I would further like to thank my friends, teachers and mentors within the counselling and therapeutic world. My retraining and development as a counsellor has been greatly assisted by their help and support. I would particularly like to mention Ellen Noonan, Gerald Wooster, John Foskett, John Boreham and Eileen Smith. I am grateful to those who have accompanied me on my journey inwards and have enabled my emotional growth. To my husband Peter Buckroyd with this book, as with others, I owe an enormous amount. Without his sustained practical help and continuing support and encouragement this book would not have been written.

J.B.
London, 1989

Preface to the Second Edition

In the five years since this book was written public interest in and awareness of eating disorders has increased enormously. A great deal of new research has been done and much has been written both for the popular and for the academic reader. One over-riding reality is clear: that the incidence of eating disorders in both the male and female populations shows absolutely no sign of decreasing. Awareness of these problems among health professionals has improved but there is still a great sense of helplessness as to how to offer any useful advice to that vast majority of sufferers whose difficulties are not so great that they come to the attention of hospitals and psychiatrists but who nevertheless are made thoroughly miserable by a way of behaving that seems impossible to change.

The first edition of this book focused on offering a range of ways to make emotional sense of an eating disorder. In this edition I have made an addition to that material. This new chapter uses the growing evidence that eating disorders have often at their root the experience of sexual abuse in childhood. No-one who works in the field of mental health can escape the knowledge that such abuse is far more common than anyone guessed only a few years ago. And since this abuse is perpetrated most often on the bodies of girls, it is not surprising that the lasting mark of it can be also a physical affliction to a woman's body.

The other major addition to the original text of this book is a section which suggests how eating disordered people can begin to engage in the emotional work that can eventually free them from the grasp of their compulsive behaviour. It is one thing (and a very major step forward) to begin to have some idea of what lies behind the problem; it is another and much longer process to work through those difficulties to the point where they begin to be less troubling. The new section of the book offers a range of exercises and activities to stimulate thinking, exploring and working through the traumas of the past and the problems of the present. Perhaps, ideally, an eating disordered person should have professional help to promote and support this process. The reality is that relatively few people find their way to counselling or therapy and that even among counsellors and therapists there are relatively few with the appropriate expertise. Self-help and support from family and friends are the best that most can hope for – and in this case the suggestions provided may be useful.

Finally the resources section of the book has been revised to take account of new publications and the changing provision of help.

My own thinking has developed considerably over this past five years. I would like to acknowledge with gratitude my working partnership with my fellow therapist, Wendy Dobbs, during this period. Together we have sought to find new and experiential methodologies for working with groups of eating disordered women. Much of what is new in this edition of the book originates in that work. I would also like to acknowledge the stimulus to thought I have gained from a Swedish dance therapist colleague and dear friend, Karin Thulin. During this time I have finished my training with the Guild of Psychotherapists and have derived much benefit from the support and encouragement of two of my teachers especially, Eleanor Armstrong Perlman and Nina Farhi. Since this book was first written I have worked with many more women including some from a wider age range than I had previously encountered. They also have helped me to develop my understanding and my capacity to be of use to them. It is to them that this second edition is affectionately dedicated.

J.B.
London, 1993

SECTION ONE

1

Eating disorders are not about food

We need to understand what a woman is saying when she uses her body to express difficult emotional issues. We need to understand why it is safer to say, 'I need to go on a diet' than 'I feel hurt or upset or in conflict.'

Susie Orbach, *Fat is a Feminist Issue*

This book is written for those who are unhappy about the way they use food. It is partly for those who find it hard to eat. Those are the people who get hungry but who don't want to eat. Perhaps they feel they can't. And there are people who would rather be thin than satisfy hunger. It is for those people especially who are afraid that they cannot eat, and afraid that the problem is out of control. And it is for those who sometimes with part of themselves would like to be able to eat and not be frightened that they will eat and eat until they are fat.

However, it is also written for those people who eat too much, those who eat when they are not hungry, when they are already full, when they no longer want or need to eat any more. It is for those people who eat all the time and hate themselves for it. And it is for those who sometimes with part of themselves would like to be able to eat only when they are hungry or when they want to eat.

This book is also for those undereaters or overeaters, starving or bingeing, who feel the terrible need to get rid of what they have put inside themselves, however much or little. Those are the people who leave the table to go to the bathroom and stick their fingers down their throats and those who give themselves laxatives, enemas or diuretics so that they force food and drink out of their systems before it can be used and absorbed by their bodies. It is for those purgers and vomiters who sometimes with part of themselves would like to be able to eat without the terrible foreknowledge that they will have to get rid of it soon afterwards.

Nor must the families and friends and helpers of all those people with eating difficulties be overlooked. There is something terrible about watching someone who is precious to you deliberately hurting and harming herself. It is even worse when you realise that the behaviour is out of control and that it causes the sufferer tremendous emotional pain. Perhaps reading this book will help them understand better what is going on with the one they love, and how best to help and support her if she decides to try and get well.

But this book is also written for those very many women who are not so fat or so thin or so preoccupied with food that it has taken over their lives, but who, from time to time, suffer episodes of anorexia or compulsive eating or bulimia. At an all-day workshop for women involved with the care of those with eating disorders, participants were asked to do an exercise designed to encourage them to reflect upon their own misuse of food. This, when you think about it, has startling implications. The assumption is that women looking after those with eating disorders will themselves have sufficient personal experience of misusing food to understand their patients' problems. Nobody objected to this assumption. Indeed many participants found it useful to reflect upon their own eating behaviour. Yet the implication is that in this (admittedly selfselected) group of professionals 100 per cent will have adequate experience of food misuse in their own lives to help them appreciate their patients' difficulties.

HOW BIG A PROBLEM IS IT?

In a study of a group of women at college, 90 per cent of the group had used 'unnatural' means of weight control over the past year. It seems that the vast majority of modern women in the Western world find themselves, from time to time, misusing food and are anxious and bothered about that fact.

Although we live in an age where eating disorders are exceedingly common, many books on the subject start off by saying that there is nothing new about all this and that problems around food have been known for a very long time. It is certainly true that throughout recorded history there have been many people, frequently but not always women, who have used and misused food to such a remarkable degree that the fact has been noted. What is new, and what this book is concerned to point out, is that eating disorders now affect a very high proportion of women.

Problems with food, with eating, and with what that implies for size, weight and shape, are now endemic in the female population in our culture. The traditional psychoanalytic response to this situation has been to identify these problems as indications of difficulties with sexuality. Feminist writers have extended this argument and have suggested that since eating disorders are overwhelmingly a female complaint, the root of the problem lies in the way women see themselves and the pressures they are under in our culture to achieve a certain size and shape. Both of these are very useful approaches and they will be discussed later in detail. However I would like to assert that the meaning of an eating disorder to any particular woman cannot be presumed, but remains to be discovered.

Increasingly I come to think that the significance of eating disorders lies in the fact that in our culture it is the symptom which has real meaning for women. What lies behind the distress signalled by eating disorders needs to be explored and will differ from woman to woman and may also differ within that person's own history. Just as hysteria was the common symptom of distress in Freud's Vienna at the end of the last century, and is now increasingly rare, so eating disorders are becoming, and perhaps have already become, an important way that contemporary women signal emotional pain.

The idea of a symptom or a mode of behaviour belonging to one gender or another is not new. Indeed 'hysteria' in Freud's patients was largely a female complaint. Depression is also a symptom which is far more common in women than in men. On the other hand, alcohol misuse, violence and delinquency are problems (and symptoms of distress as well as crimes) overwhelmingly of men. It is a commonplace that men very often turn their distress outwards and against others, while women very often turn it inwards and against themselves. Eating disorders may well be the latest way that women have found of turning their pain inwards and acting it out on themselves.

So a major concern in this book is the fact that eating disorders are extremely common, especially among women. And central to this is the argument that not only is this something new and perhaps culturally influenced, but that it is also culturally understood. It makes sense, in other words, for our society that people have eating disorders. What I want to add to that, and what has already been implied, is that eating disorders are above all not only about eating. They are a signal from ourselves to ourselves and also perhaps to anyone else who has eyes to see and ears to hear. *What* those meanings may be will be further explored later.

THE EMOTIONAL ROOT OF EATING DISORDERS

Gross disorders of size or eating behaviour have quite often been observed and noted in the past. They have been met with puzzlement, curiosity, admiration, rage and attempts at understanding. In women, anorexia has been more frequently identified. In *Holy*

Anorexia Rudolph Bell describes how in the Middle Ages what we should now understand as anorexic behaviour – self-starvation – was regarded in religious young women as a sign of holiness and asceticism. It was noticed in the seventeenth century where a sufferer was described as 'a skeleton only clad with skin', but it was not until the nineteenth century that the syndrome was recognised by the medical profession and given a name. These nineteenth-century doctors began to be certain that anorexia had an emotional basis: 'a morbid mental state . . . hysteria'. Although there have been a number of suggested physical causes for anorexia – most recently the possibility of zinc deficiency – there has also been a consistent development over the intervening century since anorexia was first diagnosed and named, of the idea that the illness has an emotional basis which demands understanding and attention. This, however, is an exceptionally difficult task and often meets with failure.

In most cases the meaning of the eating behaviour is not obvious even to the sufferer. The meanings that come most readily to mind usually prove not very helpful to understanding what is going on. Janet French was a dancer whose story was written up in the *Evening Standard Magazine* in February 1988. She had been dancing full time since the age of 11 and was obviously talented. In the face of tremendous competition she won a place in a ballet company at the age of 17. Several years later, at the age of 22, her parents noticed a severe weight loss which Janet explained to them as the result of having been told to lose weight for her dancing. She continued to lose weight and this was then explained as the result of three members of the company having been told to leave because they were overweight. In other words, the meaning that Janet was giving to her weight loss was that it was in response to the demands of the job. Keeping the job, she was implying, was worth any amount of starvation.

The difficulty about this account of her behaviour lies in the fact that it has a certain amount of truth in it. It is the case that since about the 1960s there has been a fashion for ballet dancers (and to a lesser extent dancers generally) to be extremely thin. However, it is also possible to see by reference to photographs and paintings that this is recent aesthetic preference. Undoubtedly Janet was under great pressure to keep her weight well below the norm for her age and height. In 1985, however, Janet lost her job because she had become too weak to be able to dance. Obviously, then, whatever were the reasons for her anorexia it was not simply that Janet wanted above all else to be able to dance. In the end her anorexia lost her her job. What was tragic is that it also lost her her life.

Sometimes after the event the sufferers can tell us something of what the illness meant to them. Anna developed anorexia just at the moment when several important things happened in her life: her best friend went abroad, perhaps forever; her mother had a hysterectomy; Anna herself left home for the first time to go to college. Yet none of these things seemed to lie at the root of her illness and talking about them did not help. Gradually with the support of her family and a circle of concerned helpers, she made a spontaneous recovery over a period of more than two years. When she was about to leave college after three years, she went to see the counsellor who had originally tried to help, and talked about the illness. At that distance she felt she could understand something of what had been going on. She had been a very lively and adventurous adolescent, exploring her world and experimenting with life. Her family trusted her, felt she could take care of herself, better indeed than her less adventurous sister. Anna began to get frightened. She wasn't sure that she was in control of her sexuality, of her wildness, or of her wish to experiment. Would she be able to take care of herself in the big city where her college was situated? Perhaps not. And then what would happen? Just at that moment of anxiety her mother was operated on and her best friend left. Maybe those things felt like warnings or punishments. In any case, Anna knew that she felt the urgent need to put the brakes on her development. Looking back on her anorexia she said that she felt that she had been standing still for three years. Her social life had come to an end as well as her sexual relationships. In fact she said that she hadn't been any use to anyone. But in that time something had changed. She felt able to resume her development as a person. Her need for time out was over. So for Anna there was meaning in her anorexia and it had served a vital emotional purpose, although at enormous cost.

ANOREXIA

Anorexia is the most extreme of eating disorders and the most life threatening. For that reason it has attracted a great deal of attention. The idea that its increasing commonness is new and also that it is an illness with emotional meaning was advanced several years ago by one of the most distinguished pioneers in the attempt to understand the subject, Hilde Bruch. In *The Golden Cage*, a book that has now become a classic, she put together the understanding of the subject she had gained after years of clinical experience. Bruch wrote at a time when anorexia affected young middle-class teenagers from prosperous backgrounds. Nowadays it affects women of all ages and all classes. Yet much that Bruch wrote contained the ideas that have been so much expanded since. One of her helpful contributions has been her observation that people who starve (themselves) do not behave like ordinary rational human beings. Their starvation has biological effects which make them think and behave in strange ways. In the treatment of anorexia, therefore, there must be some space for attention to the symptom as well as to its underlying cause.

In practice it is extremely difficult to get the balance right between thinking about the code message that the eating behaviour tries to convey and responding to the practical problems which the way food is being misused will create. In a way it is much easier to respond to the eating behaviour, whether anorexia or any other eating disorder. After all, there it is straight in front of us. For that reason most of this book attempts to deal with the other half of the problem: what is it that makes people use food in such painful and unhappy ways?

COMPULSIVE EATING

Compulsive eating and obesity also have a long history, just like anorexia, and similarly they are nowadays dramatically on the increase in our culture. What is more, too many anorexics have at some time been overweight for it to be likely that anorexia and obesity are totally different things. It seems much more probable that they are opposite sides of the same coin, and both of them variations on the misuse of food.

Barbara was an American college student spending some months in England on an exchange programme. The family with whom she was living gradually became aware that she was eating very little and after some weeks approached the administrator of the programme to report that as far as they knew she was eating no more than 300 calories a day. Other students had already noticed Barbara's weight loss and had reported their anxieties, so it was not long before Barbara was challenged on the subject and after a while she agreed to see a counsellor. It then became clear that what had been noticed in England was only part of the picture. Barbara's weight fluctuated all the way from 140 lbs (63 kg) when she was at home down to less than 90 lbs (40.5 kg) when she was at college. Food, eating and body size had become a continual torment for her, and one in which she no longer had any sense of her 'real' size or of how much was a good amount to eat. Her natural sense of how much she should eat had completely deserted her. At 140 lbs (63 kg) she was considerably overweight for her age and height; at 90 lbs (40.5 kg) she was considerably under.

But if we are talking about the way obesity has been noticed historically, it has usually been the fat men of history whose enormous size or enormous appetites have been recorded: the king who 'died of a surfeit of Lampreys'; King Henry VIII whose portraits and armour reveal his girth; the Prince Regent who was so fat that he was unable to climb the stairs at his little retreat at Kenwood. Then there are the fat men of literature: Falstaff, Billy Bunter; and the fat men of legend: the entries in the *Guinness Book of Records*. Again there is a strange mixture of feelings aroused by these extraordinary figures: admiration, disgust, ridicule. Perhaps even less than with anorexia is there reason sought for these extreme cases of obesity. The monstrous discomfort might in itself lead us to seek to account for this condition. Yet the reasons given are often the most trivial and unilluminating: 'I just like my food too much; I'm just made that way; it runs in the family'.

Take, for example, the fat man of what used to be the Liberal Party, Sir Cyril Smith, MP for Rochdale, the butt of endless jokes and comments, repeatedly appearing on television screens as he awkwardly levers himself out of a car or attempts to touch (or even see) his toes. Recently he suffered a heart attack and announced his intention to retire from politics. So here is a career politician forced to retire from what he evidently likes to do by his own size. There seems a clear parallel with Janet, the anorexic dancer, and equally such behaviour so defies ordinary logic that it demands an answer, a reason.

What is more, there is a huge industry built on the back of this incomprehension. Millions of pounds are spent on calorie-reduced products, on diet books, classes, regimes designed to enable people to reach or retain an ordinary size and weight. What is generally acknowledged is that virtually all of the weight lost by these systems is regained. Yet the obvious conclusion that people attain the weight they do, become the size they are, for some very good emotional meaning, is neglected. Certainly it would not be good for business if it were generally understood that buying aids to weight loss is most unlikely to be a useful or helpful thing to do. Yet I think that we should do ourselves this much credit and believe that we would not have made ourselves the shape and size we are without very good reason. Moreover, it will be obvious to many of us that any weight or size alteration is likely to be temporary unless something changes inside us.

Elizabeth Taylor, a woman who lives in the public eye if ever a woman did, has written what amounts to an autobiography of her size, weight and shape changes over the years. It is a depressing catalogue of weight lost and regained. However, eventually Elizabeth Taylor saw the light:

> But since I finally made up my mind to do something about my weight I have never wavered from my goal. The difference this time was that I was also willing to face the emotional needs behind my obesity and do something about those problems too. (*Elizabeth Takes Off*, Macmillan, 1988.)

Feminist writers think that weight loss for women is a massive con trick visited upon women by means of the advertising industry which equates thinness with sexual attractiveness and holds up unrealistic ideals for size and shape to women (and also, though they do not say so, for men). However, we would be deceiving ourselves if we did not acknowledge that there are also large numbers of overweight and obese people in our society.

It is true that some women would only feel really thin enough if they regained their prepubescent weight – a goal that, fortunately for our health, is probably unattainable for most of us. But it is also true that many women feel uncomfortable for practical reasons at the size they are and would like to lose some weight. The mystery to them is why they cannot, or why if they do they so rapidly regain the weight that they have lost. Catherine in her late thirties was considerably plumper than she wanted to be. At a time in her life when her morale was high and she felt able to be the person she wanted to be, she gradually and in a moderate and determined sort of way lost weight until she felt herself to be a comfortable size and weight. Within a year she had put it all back on again. She was amazed and angry at herself. It had taken so much determination to get the weight off; how was it that, without consciously intending to do so, she had regained it within so short a space of time? She knew better than anyone that there had to be a reason for such unsatisfying behaviour. It seems that many women in our society use being overweight as some kind of message to themselves and perhaps also to others.

BULIMIA

If anorexia and compulsive eating have long recorded histories, even though they might be infinitely more common now, what does appear to be quite new is the most painful and distressing of all eating disorders, bulimia – the bingeing and purging or vomiting that so many food misusers find their way to. No one can keep anorexia or compulsive eating a secret for all that long; the physical effects become visible to anyone who cares to look. But bulimia is the most secret, the most shameful, the most isolating and desolate of all food misuse. Its effects can be very serious physically but are rarely seen by the outsider. It remains a private torment.

WHY SOME PEOPLE MISUSE FOOD

Our concern here is to try and understand what the misuse of food, whatever form it takes, might mean to the individual. The whole of the book rests on the idea that the way we use food does have meaning, even though that meaning might be far from obvious, and not consciously known to the sufferer. It is instead of something; it is instead of feeling, or knowing, or understanding something that feels too difficult or frightening or unacceptable. It is designed to protect us from what we suspect about ourselves. Eating disorders are very preoccupying – we intend them to be; we need them to be, otherwise they would fail in their protective function. And the more frightening that hidden, unknown, suspected something is, the more resolutely we will cling on to our eating disorder. One of the terrible things about eating disorders is that it is very hard for the sufferer to believe that beginning to think and feel and understand what it might be about will not be worse than the pain of the condition itself. Often it seems as though, however painful and upsetting the eating disorder is, the prospect of reflecting upon its meaning is even more painful – in fact impossible. It is for that reason that eating disorders often go on for years and become a way of life.

What is more, it is probably true that there are some difficult things to be known or understood by the food misuser. There *is* something that needs attention, needs to be dealt with; some part of our experience, of our history, some unfinished business. It is unlikely to be very agreeable or very easy or we would not have needed to misuse food rather than let ourselves know about it. But we pay a very high price for the decision not to know. We stunt our development as people, just as Anna brought her life to a standstill with her three years of anorexia. We cheat ourselves of the human possibilities there might be for us.

Diana was a young woman brought up in conditions of extreme maltreatment and deprivation. Yet she had considerable talent as a dancer. Against all the odds she began to develop that talent but after three years of training she first developed anorexia and then bulimia. For her there were all sorts of terrible things about her past that she did not want to know. She could not keep them out of her dreams, but she could keep them out of her life during the day because she thought of nothing but food – how much, how little, when, what sort, how to get it out of her body once she had put it inside. Diana did not enjoy her eating disorder – it was a constant torment to her – but she resolutely maintained that the awful things that had happened to her, her present loneliness, her fear of people, were not important or worth thinking about. The only thing 'wrong' with her was her eating disorder. All she needed was some help with that. She got some help with that – nutritional advice, medical support – but nothing changed. She said sadly that she could not imagine ever being able to live without her preoccupation. But in the meantime so great was her absorption in the ins and outs of food and eating and weight and body size that she stopped dancing. The one really good and positive thing in her life was being destroyed.

We most of us do not have so terrible a history to deal with as Diana, nor are we so totally absorbed in our food misuse that we bring our lives to a standstill, yet even so we waste our lives and our possibilities. Emma was a capable young woman in her late twenties who held down a responsible job and lived an energetic social life. However, she was very frightened of men and found it impossible to accept offers of dates from men although she would like to have done so. Besides she had found a way of not worrying about that part of her life by worrying about her weight instead. Over a period of six years or so she steadily put on weight and was much heavier than she wanted to be. She had tried innumerable diets but had always abandoned them or put back the weight she had lost. When she began to dare to think through her feelings about men she also began to lose weight and to be freed from her preoccupation with it.

The thing about eating disorders is that they change the currency. Something that belongs to our emotional life, that is about feelings, is being expressed physically by means of behaviour. It is a symptom that simultaneously reveals and conceals. We are using a language that is difficult to translate, difficult for us and usually impossible for other people (or why would they say such things as 'I don't know why you don't eat a bit less/more/more sensibly'?). We believe somewhere inside our heads that we are protecting ourselves from something dreadful by our eating disorders; we think we have found a way of coping with what otherwise seems unmanageable. Instead we create for ourselves a much worse problem by creating a ritual behaviour whenever the world gets too frightening.

Initially the eating disorder is not the problem – we intend it to be the answer to the problem – but it can *become* the problem very quickly. After all, if you lose your job (or in some terrible cases your life) your solution to the problem is hardly brilliant. Even at a much less serious level staying at home counting calories and worrying about your weight and what you have eaten, what you are eating or what you intend to eat does not rate highly as a rewarding way to spend time.

If you suffer from eating disorders and have read thus far there is, however, something on your side, and that is your own curiosity about yourself and a certain amount of motivation to live your life differently. This book is an attempt to help you think about what it might be that you are trying to express or hide or otherwise deal with by means of your eating behaviour. If there were not a part of you willing to try, you would not have got this far. That is not to say that getting better and changing is an easy matter. It is not, for any of us. We all have very mixed feelings about giving up what has become our way of doing things. But at the very beginning I said that this book was for people who are unhappy about the way they use food. You have that on your side to help you – your creative discontent with the way you do things at the moment.

Of course we can all postpone changing. We can hope that things will get better all by themselves without us having to put any thought or effort into making it happen. Most of us long for a magic wand which will change the way things are for us. Unfortunately there are no magic wands and sooner or later we have to take responsibility for the way we live our lives. Sadly if we don't want to get better, at least with a bit of us, nobody can make us. As Anna said when she thought about her three years of anorexia: 'While I didn't want to get better, it didn't matter what anyone said.'

What do you think of when you think of food?

One day in winter, on my return home, my mother, seeing that I was cold, offered me some tea, a thing I did not ordinarily take . . . She sent for one of those squat, plump little cakes called 'petites madeleines', which look as though they have been moulded in the fluted valve of a scallop shell. And soon . . . I raised to my lips a spoonful of the tea in which I had soaked a morsel of the cake. No sooner had the warm liquid mixed with the crumbs touched my palate than a shudder ran through me and I stopped, intent upon the extraordinary thing that was happening to me. An exquisite pleasure had invaded my senses, something isolated, detached with no suggestion of its origin . . .

And suddenly the memory revealed itself. The taste was that of the little piece of madeleine which on Sunday mornings at Combray . . . my aunt Leonie used to give me, dipping it first in her own cup of tea . . .

And as soon as I had recognised the taste of the piece of madeleine . . . (although I did not yet know and must long postpone the discovery of why this memory made me so happy) immediately the old grey house upon the street, where her room was, rose up like a strange set . . . and the good folk of the village and their little dwellings and the parish church and the whole of Combray and its surroundings, taking shape and solidity, sprang into being, town and gardens alike, from my cup of tea.

Marcel Proust, *Remembrance of Things Past*

Although I have stressed the fact that eating disorders are not about food and that I am concerned to explore what lies behind them, yet it is important to pay some attention to why we might choose this way of expressing our inner selves. For each of us food and eating have a long history and a lifetime of meaning. We can probably begin to find some clues about why we use food in the way we do in the story of our experience of it. In this chapter I want to trace some of our memories of and associations to food during the course of our development. Your part in this process is to recreate your own history and see if you can glimpse some of the inner logic behind your use of food now.

EARLY EXPERIENCES OF FOOD

Good feeding experiences as babies are important because they leave us with memory traces of blissful states which we may later try to recapture. We come into the world totally dependent on our caregivers for our life to continue, but also the vast majority of us are ready to play our part by being able and willing to suck. The baby is hungry, the food appears, the baby sucks and is satisfied. There are some mothers and babies for whom it is that simple some of the time. Perhaps for most of us there are some times when it is that easy, that good. The image of a satisfied, contented baby going off to sleep in its mother's arms is a powerful symbol of total happiness, total security. Maybe for most of us there is some residual memory of blissful fullness and physical comfort.

However, for many the early experiences of food, of hunger, of eating, are not always or even often very straightforward. It takes confidence to feed a tiny baby well, and in our western culture mothers are often not very confident. We have, for instance, became so anxious about our ability to feed our babies from our own breasts that the *majority* of us do not even try to do so. The reason we give is that we do not know how much the baby is getting. We would rather trust a bottle full of reconstituted modified cows' milk than what we ourselves produce.

There is also the fact that we do not always match the baby's need for food soon enough, quickly enough, accurately enough to prevent distress, and it is now half a century since it was first recognised by Melanie Klein what agony that sense of acute hunger arouses in the baby. Hunger is something it cannot name, cannot understand or account for, but only suffer. And that suffering probably induces panic, terror, a violent physical experience perhaps like being torn apart. Most of us adults have experienced hunger acute enough to cause us pain, maybe even panic, but we have a whole world of understanding into which to fit those feelings and with which to help us cope with them. The baby has no such containing framework.

Very few of us can consciously remember those early feeding experiences. We want to believe that they have no effect on us, but it seems very likely that the intensity of that feeding experience remains with us in some preconscious, non-verbal way. For those who misuse food these earliest experiences may well be one element in later difficulties. Charlene had been among those babies who actually experienced starvation. Her mother was simply not equal to the fierce demands of looking after a baby. Charlene was kept alive with ice lollies, until at six months she was taken from her mother and put into care. As a young adult Charlene became a compulsive eater who was never full enough, never satisfied.

Of course, that is not the whole story. A baby's experience of being fed is also the experience of being loved, held, taken care of, protected. Missing out on one means missing out on the other experiences too. Charlene's compulsive eating was not only the endless attempt to undo the real physical neglect twenty years earlier, but also the attempt to repair the emotional hurt and damage. It is easy to see in this case how hopeless an enterprise that was; perhaps Charlene's hurts could be healed by better experience of being loved, but certainly they could not be healed by compulsive eating.

For some of us, of a certain generation, there was the difficulty that our mothers were taught to disregard their natural urges to pick us up and feed us when we cried and were hungry. Truby King was the male author of manuals of infant care who urged mothers to believe that it was actually harmful for babies to be fed at other than strict four-hourly intervals, however much they cried, and that babies should not be handled more than strictly necessary. The suffering of a sensitive mother who believed such nonsense is surely equal only to the suffering of the baby who received such treatment. These babies must have the most terrible early physical and emotional experience of the pangs of hunger.

Another major event in our infant experience of feeding is weaning. There is so much conflicting advice and so many pressures on mothers now that it is exceedingly difficult for them to attend to the baby's development and to select the right moment for a move away from milk to solids. Some mothers breastfeed for the six weeks that it is said that human milk conveys antibodies to the child and then switch to a bottle with solids. Some give milk for the six months that the baby's natural iron supplies are said to last and then introduce solids. Some read what has been said about the possibility of triggering gluten allergy by feeding cereals too soon and begin solid feeding with puréed fruit and so on. Many mothers return to work after six weeks maternity leave and that necessarily puts an end to breastfeeding if not to bottle feeding.

Very few mothers have the freedom — practical or emotional — and the confidence to wait and see what their baby wants and needs and when it will happily, and with curiosity and pleasure, begin to explore the interesting possibilities of mixed feeding. For many babies the weaning process may feel like something frightening and depriving; something known and good is being taken away and being replaced by something strange and difficult and unpleasant. The sweet milk (and it is remarkable just how sweet breast milk is; cows' milk has sugar added to it as part of the process of modifying it for babies) is replaced by an alien texture and taste.

It seems likely that these early feeding experiences lead to various sorts of food misuse. One is the feeling of not being able to rely on there being food again – the need to eat to satiety now because the opportunity will not come again. An echo of weaning, perhaps, lies in the preference of many food misusers for foods that are sweet and easy to eat, requiring little chewing. Could this be why fast food chains such as MacDonalds are so successful and why so many people like ice cream and soft drinks? Maybe a lot of us learned to doubt and misunderstand our feelings of hunger. Probably most of us did not have enough of that early experience of breast/bottle feeding and we find culturally approved ways of making up for ourselves for the nasty shock of it being brought to an end so soon.

There is a great deal more to eating disorders than the attempt to reverse or recreate early feeding experience, but the central importance of that experience in our infant lives makes it worth considering and investigating. If you want to think about your misuse of food, it might be worth trying to explore that subject by talking to those who knew you as a baby. Perhaps you can learn something about the roots of your present difficulties in that early history.

FOOD AS PART OF AN EARLY POWER STRUGGLE

However, the meaning of food and eating does not only derive from our infant experience. We have a whole lifetime of personal meanings to add to those beginnings.

The next in chronological order, and one that may well be within reach of conscious memory for some of us, is the battle that is often conducted over food with toddlers and young children. We have all heard adults say with mingled amounts of pride, despair and annoyance about young children, 'Oh, she's got a mind of her own.' Children naturally develop the capacity to want, whether it is the rattle held out to them in earliest infancy or the more sophisticated playthings and experiences of later childhood. In this wanting lies the kernel of our capacity to grow into adults who will be able to make good choices for ourselves and for our lives. Parents often find this wanting hard to deal with anyway, and can feel challenged by a child's capacity to want differently from its parents. It is difficult, and probably impossible, to get right the balance between allowing children freedom to choose and appropriately limiting their choices, especially as the territory is always moving anyway. It is easy to offer a 2-year-old the choice between milk and juice, but what about the 8-year-old who wants coffee or the 12-year-old who wants beer?

Unfortunately it is often food which is chosen as the battleground on which the child's struggle for separation and independence is worked out. And these issues are complicated by the meanings of food and feeding as loving and caring that were referred to in connection with infant feeding. Parents, especially mothers, can have too much invested in getting their child to eat everything up. Not eating can too easily be seen as rejection of what has been offered and therefore of the one who offers it. I remember reading advice to mothers not to take too much time or trouble over preparing darling little meals for tiny children. If the child spits out what you have taken hours to make, you are much more likely to be upset than if it took you ten minutes and/or (perish the thought) you opened a packet or a tin. It seems an appropriate acknowledgement of the fact that it's easy for mothers to feel rejected and upset over children's eating behaviour, and easy to be emotionally over-invested in whether the little one eats her egg.

In this sense of rejection lie the roots of the anger and the power struggle that so frequently follow a child's refusal of food. Of course parents can justify anger by reference to what they think are the child's needs, yet it is widely known and understood that there is a time in the lives of young children when their need for food diminishes sharply. We also know because we have read it a hundred times that if a child is normal in every other way and full of energy, then however little food she gets it is enough. This truth can be hard to hang on to when all your child will eat is peanut butter sandwiches, but it is sometimes reassuring.

Despite this we nevertheless try and force children to eat. Why? Perhaps it has something to do with the unpalatable fact that as parents it is our function to become unnecessary. In the first intimation of the fact that our child is capable of not wanting what we want is the distant trumpet call that sounds the end of our usefulness in that role. Our violence in reinforcing our will is the measure of how hard it is for us to endure that hard fact.

Often people write as though the difficulties over children's eating behaviour were only to do with the child. It is also very much to do with the parent. An authority on psychological matters was writing about how children have to learn to deal with frustration. He (it was a man) suggested that it was appropriate to make children finish food and to eat food they did not like in order to accustom them to frustration. This quite remarkably stupid advice reveals an author apparently unaware of the many, many necessary frustrations in a child's everyday life. To advocate adding food to the list not only sets the stage for endless battles, but lays the foundations for trouble in the future.

Two adults, Gordon and Hilda, both in their fifties, were discussing their experience with food as children. Hilda told how as a child she was required to eat everything put in front of her, whether she liked it or not, and whether she was hungry or not. If she would not eat it she was given nothing else to eat and at each meal what she had not previously eaten was put in front of her until she did. Such brutal and humiliating ways of dealing with children are perhaps not quite as common these days. Gordon then told how he was allowed to eat what he wanted. At one time for a while he ate nothing but bananas and orange juice. At this point in the story Hilda, his wife, interrupted to say how very spoiled and indulged he had been as a child. The interesting thing is that one of these adults is what is called a 'picky eater' and dislikes a great many foods. The other is a curious and adventurous eater and will try anything. I will leave you to work out which is which.

Once the power struggle is located in food, then both parties are likely to play the game with great enthusiasm and persistence. That is bad enough in itself, but there is worse to follow. It seems that often the struggle we carried on in reality as small children with our parents, we continue as grown people in our heads. We install the parent figure inside us. We internalise her (him, them) and we continue to respond to this internal parent as we responded, or wanted to respond, to the real parent.

Isobel came from a family where food was in short supply. This was not because there was any lack of money but because Isobel's mother believed in strictly limiting portions of food. She always bought the absolute minimum quantities of everything and never kept any supplies in the cupboard. Each day's food was bought a day at a time and there were no extras to allow for unexpected changes or snacks. So there were never any biscuits or any 'instant food' for peckish moments.

Isobel had coped with this mean and depriving household as best she could – because, of course, what went with it was a mother who felt that her emotional resources were in as short supply as the food and who found it impossible to respond with generosity to the emotional hunger of her family. As a child Isobel found substitute mothers in her teachers and the families of her friends and then from her mid-teens in sexual relationships with boys considerably older than herself from whom she could get some 'mothering'. This system broke down when she left her home town to go to college. There she began to eat voraciously, eating to fill the void of unlovedness, but also to defy the mother who practised such rigid portion control. To eat a whole packet of biscuits became an act of hatred and revenge against the mother who now in reality was quite unable to limit Isobel's consumption.

WOMEN AND FOOD – THE DILEMMA

This account of Isobel and her mother makes clear another aspect of food use which is particularly difficult for women. This is that mothers (girlfriends, wives, sisters) are often the ones who do the preparing of food, the shopping and cooking, but are also the ones required to limit their food intake. Feminists have made us aware of the cultural requirement for women to be thin. As they have pointed out, virtually all women's magazines will contain sections on food restriction for women ('The Three Day Diet'; 'Get your Body Ready for the Beach', etc.). Side by side with these instructions will be others urging them to feed their families ('Hearty Puddings for your Family'; 'Scrumptious Casseroles for Hungry Males', etc.). The apparent requirement is that we starve ourselves while urging others to eat ('Go on, eat it up; it'll do you good.').

This complex message about how to deal with food in relation to our families is paralleled by what is often understood by women as the demand to take care of everyone else and not to take care of themselves. Women are to be generous with others emotionally, take care of their needs and wants, but ignore their own needs. This painful dynamic – and the transmission of it from mother to daughter – has been described by Susie Orbach and others. These cultural messages make it extremely hard for women to know whether they are allowed to eat, or certainly what and how much. Many of the women I talked to said they had an index in their heads of forbidden foods – forbidden, that is, to them, but not to others. Food is made to do the work of all kinds of complicated feelings about loving and not loving.

THE ROLE OF FOOD IN THE FAMILY

This brings us to another dimension of our experience of food and eating. We have been talking so far about the relationship between mother (or primary caregiver) and child in relation to food. Although that is an extremely important dimension of our experience, it is only part of it. There is the whole issue of the meaning of food in our family. What were food and mealtimes used for in our households?

The Jardine family were noisy, boisterous and numerous. Their mealtimes were times of exuberant conversation during which they competed with one another for conversational space. They kept open house and the children's friends frequently came and joined in these highspirited occasions. Kate, their mother, was an exceptionally good cook and produced, apparently without undue effort, large quantities of good food. Leonard, their father, was a supportive and appreciative husband who frequently thanked his wife for the excellent food that all of them had just enjoyed. For the Jardine mealtimes were joyful opportunities for celebration. This is not to say that they did not have their sorrows or their quarrels, but mealtimes were often happy occasions.

Interestingly enough the Jardines were all slightly overweight, as if the pleasure of eating and mealtimes was too good to resist, but none of them appeared to mind. Perhaps this can support what I am trying to say about the use of food. If you use food to celebrate as the Jardines did and in the process get rather plump, that is only an issue if it makes you unhappy. If you enjoy the way you use food, there is no problem. This is where I agree with the feminist writers who have urged women to let themselves find out what size and shape they want to be regardless of what the advertising industry holds up for admiration.

The Knight family, on the other hand, had dismal and frightening mealtimes. The father of the family, Malcolm, was a violent and evil-tempered man who terrorised his wife Nora and their children. Mealtimes were the times when he chose to pick on his family for their table manners, their clothes, what they said or the way they said it, the expression on their faces, anything or nothing. Many, many mealtimes ended with violent rages from Malcolm and tears from one or other of the family. The daughter of the family, Olivia, dealt with this situation by spending as much time as possible away from home. When she had to be part of the family she would often eat very quickly, as did her brother, apparently in an attempt to bring the meal to an end as soon as possible.

Sometimes, however, the tension made it hard for her to eat and she would have times of eating very little.

As an adult Olivia found herself repeating exactly this pattern. Tension, distress, upset would provoke either a lot of rapid and rather uncontrolled eating or an anorexic episode during which she would eat very little. It was exceedingly difficult for her to establish a regular, normal pattern of eating, and her weight fluctuated accordingly.

Patrick was brought up by his elderly grandparents. They were devoted to him but continued a pattern of existence that had been established for years and into which, as a late and unexpected arrival on the scene, he was never really integrated. Throughout his schooldays he ate alone. He would come home from school in the middle of the day or after school and would be given his meal to eat alone. There would be nothing wrong with the food but Patrick always found it difficult to concentrate on eating it. He said that he always felt as if he wanted to be out playing with his friends. His grandmother did not keep him company while he ate; it was an occasion without any kind of emotional attraction. Patrick found it extremely difficult to force himself to eat when he moved away from home. His weight was well below normal and he experienced a continual revulsion from food. However, when he began to form close relationships and to discover the pleasure of shared meals he began to be alive to how he had been continuing his family tradition with his solitary reluctant eating.

Roberta lived alone with her mother who was a nurse and worked on night shift. She had a close and even rather clinging relationship with her mother, and very few friends, so that she was accustomed to spending her evenings at home. When she came in her mother had already left for work so Roberta made her own supper and ate it in front of the television. She was lonely and hungry for her mother, but she disguised these facts from herself by turning on the television and spending the evening comforting herself with food. As she said, 'I just sit in front of the television and never notice how much I'm putting in my mouth.'

Mr and Mrs Simpson, an elderly couple, lived a life that was very unstimulating and boring. They were disappointed in life generally, which seemed to them to have been a series of hazards and crises only narrowly avoided. They saw the world outside their front door as full of danger, so they felt safer at home, living a limited but reliable routine. In this routine food assumed great importance: the planning, shopping, cooking, eating and clearing up occupied a large part of the day and their energies. This process had been going on for many years so that Mrs Simpson had steadily eaten herself to a mountainous size. In order to control the resulting hypertension, heart disease and numerous other side effects of her weight, she took large quantities of drugs which in turn produced unpleasant side effects of their own. But to the doctor's suggestion that she lose weight she responded only that she was too old, that it didn't matter, and that in any case she ate very little. 'After all,' she remarked to her husband, 'what else is there to live for?'

Mealtimes serve very different purposes in different households and form part of our experience of food. None of these examples may exactly match your own experience, but perhaps thinking about them will enable you to identify what mealtimes were for you in your family and whether you are continuing, or want to continue, that pattern and tradition.

However, food also has a meaning in families over and above the meaning of mealtimes. Deprivation of food, for example, is commonly used as a punishment. It can be an experience which lasts a lifetime. A woman in her fifties told me over and over again the story of the supper party held by her parents to which the children of the family were allowed to come. She as the youngest child was indulged when she began to entertain the company, hut her tricks went on too long, her charm ceased to amuse and her entertainment ended in her being sent to bed without any supper. At a distance of fifty years that punishment still had power to sting.

A much younger woman, Antonia, had considerably harsher treatment to deal with. Her mother had died when she was only 8 years old and her father was emotionally very ill-equipped to take care of four small children, of whom Antonia was the eldest. His methods of dealing with them were extremely unpleasant. Starvation was one of them. For trivial (or not so trivial) offences Antonia would be locked in her room for days. Only her father's wealth and position in the community protected him from prosecution for ill-treatment of his children. Antonia was unable to deal with food in a relaxed way. As a child she had stolen food, both at home where it was kept under lock and key, and from shops. A severe but short-lived anorexic few months at the age of 16 and 17 were followed by several years of very troubled eating behaviour. For a while things would be all right and then Antonia would he tormented by the urge to binge.

Perhaps more commonly than deprivation of food being used as a punishment, food can be used as a comfort. Many mothers comfort their children when they fall down with a sweet. Dentists have mostly turned to comforting their young patients with balloons rather than sweets, but doctors still hand out a sweet or a lollipop after an injection. Perhaps it is no wonder that we even have a phrase 'comfort eating' to describe this kind of consolation. And the 'comfort' for grown people is not so much for physical hurts as for emotional pain, not so much for hurt knees as for hurt feelings.

And of course food is used as a reward and as a bribe. Sometimes when I have worked with people with eating disorders we have together devised reward systems to help them achieve changes in their eating behaviour. One of the great difficulties has been for these clients to find rewards for themselves which were *not* food. This is the cluster of feelings so accurately identified in the advertisement for cream cakes: 'Naughty but nice'. We are so thoroughly caught up in this way of seeing food that we give it all kinds of meanings. Two women were chatting at a social occasion when they were offered pieces of 'millionaire's shortbread',

shortbread covered with toffee and then with chocolate. One woman refused it on the grounds that it was immoral. Shortbread, she said, should not be covered with all that stuff. It was bad enough on its own but with topping like that it was morally offensive. Her companion, taking a piece, said that it was impossible for a biscuit to have moral value. A biscuit could not be good or bad. Can it?

The reward/bribe system works at a number of levels in our society. Business circles use it a great deal. Directors' dining rooms, expense account lunches and dinners, Christmas parties for the staff: these are all part of it. In fact, eating and food have become so important in our society that they confer status and importance. And of course where food is plentiful, as it is in our society, then all kinds of subtle meanings become attached to what is eaten when. We are none of us immune to all of this. The immense number of opportunities to eat, the endless attempts to titillate our jaded palates with new combinations or new ideas all combine to push us further and further away from the capacity to listen to our bodies' needs and supply them appropriately.

Take, for example, the confectionery industry's attempts to get us to use their products. They present us with the most extravagant rewards and associations to tempt us to put into our bodies something which has no nutritional value, indeed something which may well rob our bodies of nutrients. It is indicated to us that we will be socially and sexually successful. We will be beautiful. We will be young. We will be rich and leisured. Many of us are not able to resist these blandishments. That is what is intended and hoped for.

CURRENT PATTERNS OF EATING

It is now more than 40 years since the end of the Second World War, but in our (Western European) society there are still large numbers of people who remember rationing. It is now a nutritionist's commonplace to say that rationing was the best thing that ever happened to Britain because it obliged people to eat in a relatively healthy way. It was, however, not a matter of choice. As anyone will tell you who remembers those times, nobody got fat during rationing. There was a strict limit on calorie intake imposed by scarcity.

If we think about the time before the Second World War we are talking about times before the advent of the Welfare State, before the increased prosperity that we enjoy now, and when there was widespread poverty and acute hunger. There were great inequalities in society, and certainly not everyone went hungry or anything like it, but food was not as plentiful in the sense of being within the financial reach of all.

It is, then, only in the last thirty years or so that our society has been as glutted with food as it is now, and that consequently the pressures to eat have become as enormous as they are. Take a couple of small examples. Thirty years ago it was uncommon to see people eating and drinking on the streets and in public places. Now it is commonplace. Similarly, not so long ago eating between meals, even if it was a common enough activity, was thought to be a bad idea. Now for increasing numbers of people there are no established mealtimes and changes in the food industry have eroded established patterns of what to eat. The phenomenon known as 'grazing' is upon us where it is normal to eat all day long in an unstructured way and without much reference to time of day. The old certainties of how much of what to eat when are disappearing. For those of us whose inner psychological certainty about food has been damaged, the trackless territory of contemporary eating behaviour creates tremendous problems. Interestingly enough, programmes for recovering food misusers often include a requirement to eat in a thoroughly conventional way at fixed mealtimes, so that in one dimension at least there is some guidance.

Some Western European countries – perhaps France, Spain,

Italy, maybe others – seem to the casual observer at least to have suffered less disintegration in family structures than Britain or the USA. In these countries meals seem a much more important family occasion and to have retained formal and ritual value. This may, perhaps, help those who otherwise might lose their bearings completely about food and hunger.

Quite apart from the personal and inner difficulties with food, society as a whole has not adapted well to the constant availability and abundance of food. So far as I know, no society has. North America has had to deal with the situation longer than Western Europe; the difficulties this created started earlier and chart a path that it looks as if we are following.

However, it could only be in a society in which food was so immensely important that eating disorders would make sense. This is very obviously the case with anorexia. To put it crudely: if you are anorexic in a society in which many people are underfed then you are not so remarkable, but to starve in a society of overfed people is something very different. This is equally true of obesity. In a society where food is in short supply, then to be fat is a signal of the power to choose to eat when that power is not general. It therefore conveys wealth or status within the society. Where we all have the opportunity to overeat, the fact that only some take it gives that gesture emotional meaning and significance. If, even more strangely, people eat and then get rid of the food so that it cannot nourish them, they make an even more violent statement.

This chapter has shown how our personal experience and the society in which we live supply us with a context for our eating behaviour. This experience does not necessarily turn us into food misusers, but it does give us a language, a way of behaving, if we get to the point of feeling that we have to use it. It gives us weapons, ammunition of a certain kind, if we need to take them up. What I now want to go on to explore is what reasons there might be for us taking up these very powerful weapons.

SECTION TWO

3

Eating disorders as a response to crisis

This [behaviour in crisis] was a temporary hitch in a reasonably well-managed life.

Ellen Noonan, *Counselling Young People*

In the first section we looked at the emotional meaning of the use of food, food misuse. Let us now consider it as a response to crisis. Take this very mild and very common example: a young woman goes out to a party or for a meal. She eats far more than she wants to and comes home feeling angry that she has not exerted more self-control. She asks herself why she did it and produces a range of answers that sound possible, but not convincing: she had to eat not to offend her hostess; she was just greedy and lost control; she didn't notice that she was eating too much; she particularly liked the food and couldn't resist eating too much. But if we explore a little more carefully what this young woman was feeling before she went to the party we discover that there was a mixture of feelings about it, not all of which were very easy to deal with. Yes, she was looking forward to it, but she also felt anxious about it. Who would she meet? What would people think of the way she looked or danced? Perhaps she also felt sexually excited and couldn't feel very contented or relaxed with that feeling. Perhaps with a part of her she didn't want to go to the party at all, felt resentful and angry because she would have preferred to do something else.

There could be any number of feelings associated with a social event of this kind and feelings that are difficult for one person will be pleasurable for another. The point is that for some women one way of dealing with those difficult feelings is to smother them with food. Now this may be the way some women have developed of dealing with difficult feelings. In this chapter, however, I'm suggesting that it can be the way some women respond to crisis, to a particular situation, that for them feels particularly difficult.

There is, of course, no good reason why a woman should abandon this way of coping if it causes her no pain. After all, if she occasionally eats too much or doesn't eat enough as a way of dealing with a crisis, no great harm has been done. We all need some defences and that one may be as good as any. However, some women don't like the way they use food, are bothered by it, don't understand it, and would like to change, and it is to them that this is directed.

We use our emergency ways of coping when we feel most under stress or threat. One of the commonest and most obvious of these situations is when a girl leaves home for the first time. Very often this move to college or to her own place is accompanied by a quite considerable weight gain or loss. This is such a frequent occurrence that there is a whole series of common sense reasons that are produced to explain it: the food in the hostel is stodgy; she doesn't like the food they give her; she's eating too much fast food instead of cooking for herself; she's not eating a balanced diet; she doesn't know how to cook properly; the cooking facilities aren't very good; she has to share the kitchen with so many other people; she's a vegetarian and the hostel gives her such boring vegetarian food – and so on.

Yet it seems that for many young people, leaving home for the first time is an especially difficult moment in their lives. It doesn't help that it is probably something they wanted to do with a size-able chunk of themselves, that they were thoroughly fed up with living at home and very conscious of its problems and disadvantages. They expected to be able to make a painless transition into independent living and very probably other people expected it of them too: 'You'll be looking forward to getting a place of your own . . . I expect you're looking forward to doing your own thing . . . You'll be glad to get away to college.' Of course, for many there are these feelings, but they are not as simple and unmixed as other people seem to expect, or as they expect of themselves.

What is being referred to here is the ordinary anxiety about transition from being an adolescent living at home to being a young adult establishing her own independence. It does not refer to the much more serious difficulties to be discussed later of those eating disorders that are the effect of serious and long-standing problems in making the transition from child to adolescent to adult. However, because these more short-lived difficulties are not so serious, it does not mean that they are not painful.

FIONA'S STORY

Fiona got herself a place at a college in London a long way from her family home. Her family lived in a quiet, remote part of the country and there lived a quiet, rather old-fashioned and conservative life. Fiona was herself a rather quiet, conservative, old-fashioned girl. However, she obviously, with part of herself at least, wanted something more exciting or she would never have contemplated so radical a move. The reality of living and going to college in London was horrifying to her. She was appalled by the way her fellow students spoke and behaved. She was shocked by their bad language and their sexually explicit conversations. She was threatened by their active sexuality, by the self-confidence, as she saw it, the pushiness, of some of the students. She felt there was almost no one like her and her obvious disapproval and contempt for her fellow students certainly did not help her to make friends. She could survive in an alienated kind of way while she was actually at college, but when she went home she fell apart.

And the band-aid that she chose to cover her wounds with was food. Evening after evening she would sit on her own in the deserted kitchen of the hostel eating bread and butter, for her the symbolic food of childhood and of home. By half-term she had gained a stone in weight and lost a ton in confidence and self-esteem. She suffered worst from agonies of home-sickness and it was this feeling in particular that she tried to anaesthetise with food. With dogged courage she stuck out most of the first year of her course. It was only when she began to accept that it was no disgrace to be homesick that she could allow herself to consider other courses and other colleges nearer home.

There was nothing wrong with Fiona's development as an adolescent, but she had made a change that was more than she was ready for at the time. When she could feel that she need not be ashamed of her feelings, she did not need to try to obliterate them with bread and butter but instead could begin to make plans that were more appropriate to her temperament and her emotional development.

ALISTAIR'S STORY

A young man, Alistair, came to college in London from a background not unlike Fiona's: quiet, conservative and provincial. He, however, was bursting to get away and longing to sample what London had to offer. Almost immediately, however, he began to lose weight so rapidly and to such an extent that he looked for some help. What emerged was a story of an extremely capable and energetic young man who at the same time was deeply resentful that now he was no longer living at home there was no one to look after him and he had to look after himself. At a practical level the adult part of Alistair was more than capable of doing this, but the child part wanted a mother to take care of him, particularly to cook for him. When there was no one, the hurt and angry child part of him responded by not eating. Now on top of this dynamic there was a whole layer of apparent reasons why Alistair hadn't been eating: there wasn't time to shop or cook; his grant was late so he had no money; he didn't know how or what to cook and so on. Nevertheless, although there was truth in all of this, the guts of the situation was that Alistair wasn't eating because he was so upset and angry about leaving home (and what home meant – having his meals provided for him). When he could accept that there was a bit of him that felt like that, and that his grief and upset at leaving home was usual and normal, then he could begin to enjoy his independence and take pleasure in becoming a very competent cook.

TIME TO MOURN

In both of these situations there had been some emotional work left undone, very possibly emotional work for which there was no encouragement or opportunity for these two people. And that emotional work is the work of grieving. Most of us think about our lives as progress (at least to middle age) towards something better. The advantages of being older and more grown up than in fact we are appear constantly before our eyes. This applies not only to the natural urge for physical mastery and maturity – co-ordination, physical strength, height, weight – but also in adolescents to social mastery. The freedoms to smoke, drink, stay up late, go out without adults, have sexual experience, see adult films, earn more money: these are very seductively displayed and make it difficult sometimes for us to allow ourselves to be the age we are emotionally and chronologically. One effect of this, then, is that it is hard to mourn for the pleasures of the part of our life that we are leaving behind. Peter Pan gets very little sympathy these days, yet I suspect there are few of us who entered puberty and adolescence without a pang for what we were leaving behind.

There is a similar story to be told at the point of transition from adolescence to young adulthood. To express sadness at leaving home – sadness that a whole part of our life with our parents is over – is not always very easy. The cultural climate does not encourage it. But nevertheless the evidence is that such natural mourning is not an optional extra but a necessary and desirable part of our capacity to take up the challenges of the next stage of our development.

FOOD AND RELATIONSHIPS

Another area of crisis is that of relationships. It is very common for women who use food in crisis to binge or starve when relationships go wrong – especially love relationships. Again it is the ordinary ups and downs that are part of the process of looking for a long-term partner that are being talked about here, not the more serious eating disorders (to be discussed later) where those who find it exceedingly difficult to form relationships at all may use eating disorders as a holding pattern to keep the whole issue at a distance. However, the 'ordinariness' of such crises in no way diminishes their capacity to cause a lot of pain.

Take, for example, the story of Iris, a lively, clever, funny, popular girl who lived an extremely busy, active social life. One of the reasons she was so popular was that she was always good-tempered, always smiling. When she split up with her boyfriends, she didn't feel it bothered her. She got a bit upset, that was all: easy come, easy go. Her sadness soon passed and she was her old self again.

But underneath this jolly coping self was a girl who dealt with the crises with the men in her life by eating. This fact she kept secret from herself for a long time, although she was upset by her inability to keep her weight down. She did not know in any sort of conscious way what she was doing. Anyway, this system had worked not badly for about three years, so why should she know? But one autumn she broke up with a boy whom she had been very fond of. Her weight increased. She began not to cope at work. She started taking a lot of time off and became depressed. Depression was something new in her life. She had, as far as she could remember, never felt so miserable before. It was sufficiently alarming for her to seek help, particularly because, as she said, nothing was wrong in her life. She didn't know what she was depressed about. So far as she was concerned it had just happened to her.

Gradually, as she began to try to remember when she got depressed and what had been happening in her life at that time, it became obvious to her that she had been upset by the break-up with her boyfriend. But that was a puzzle to her because she didn't get upset about boyfriends. Then, without recognising the connection, Iris began to talk about the real problem in her life: her failure to control her weight and eating. Soon she began to see the connection. Maybe she didn't consciously get upset, but certainly something was hurting inside when she stuffed herself with food. Then we began to talk about her family and how they dealt with crisis. The answer was that they didn't. No one was allowed to get upset, particularly not Iris. Her mother insisted that Iris always presented a smiling face and had been known to hang up on her if her telephone calls were not sufficiently up-beat.

In fact, Iris's problems with food were quite an ingenious way of dealing with distress that she had never learned to express more openly. However, it was a system that had not proved strong enough to cope with a really painful loss. Her pain had emerged as depression. How was she going to do it differently?

There were lots of things going for Iris. One was that, although she had a family and a mother who had difficulties in dealing with crisis, she was fortunate that her childhood had nevertheless had lots of good things about it. She was a much-loved and cared for child. So she was not as a young woman in crisis trying to deal with a not very good beginning, as so many of those to be described in this book have had to do. If you like, all she needed was to be helped to find a way to respond more directly to her relationships with men. Secondly, she badly wanted to be rid of her problems with food. She wanted to lose weight and become as beautiful as undoubtedly she would be. She was tired of fighting herself about food all the time. So she was well-motivated to try a different way of doing it. Thirdly, although she was scared of feeling her pain, she was not very, very scared. Somewhere inside her there was a very strong, capable person (carefully nurtured by her parents) who was tough enough to survive a lot.

When we had reached this point in our discussions, I didn't see Iris for several weeks. When she came back she told me this story. She had been going on a trip with a boy who was a close friend. They were looking for the place they wanted to visit, but by mistake took a wrong turning in the car. The anxiety and frustration of the situation made Iris cry, and once started she found it hard to stop. Her friend asked her how he could help and she told him that she wanted him to take her home to his flat. This he did and he stayed with her, taking care of her. She cried for almost three days, over all the things she had not cried about for three years. She said that during those three days she had realised what a lot she had not felt and how much feeling there was to do. She said that it had been awful and terrible, but in a positive kind of way, and that she had felt incredibly much better since.

One of the remarkable things about this story is how, once given permission, Iris knew exactly what she needed to do. What's more, she could find the time and the occasion, the safe person and the safe place. Without consciously planning it, she had supplied herself with a very good opportunity to catch up on her backlog of emotional work.

Undoubtedly this is not the end of the story. Human beings don't change as fast as that. However, there has been a remarkable shift in Iris's ability to express her feelings directly. With support and encouragement there is a good chance of a lasting change. At the same time Iris's eating disorder has shrunk from being a monster to being a tendency that she knows about. When Iris wants to overeat these days, she is beginning to he able to stop and ask herself the question: 'What's upsetting me today?'

Exactly the same mechanism at work with Iris is acted out with people whose tendency is to anorexia rather than to compulsive eating. When things go badly in their intimate relationships, they starve themselves. This is not to be confused with the loss of appetite that goes with grief and mourning. The anorexia is *instead* of grief and mourning; it actually prevents any grieving and mourning. Grieving and mourning is an acknowledgement of emotional needs, hungers, dependencies, a process by which it is possible to come to terms with loss. It is that pain of need and loss that not eating is intended to abolish.

DEALING WITH ANGER

A third category of crisis to which women respond with food misuse is anger. It may seem a strange idea that anger is itself a crisis, but many women have no idea what to do with their hatred and rage, except to express it in ways that hurt themselves. On the face of it, lots and lots of women with minor eating disorders are unhappy, miserable, powerless. When women talk to me about themselves they often tell me a terrible story in which, however, no anger or outrage is expressed at all. But sometimes I know that there is rage because I feel it myself physically in my chest. Suddenly I will feel furiously angry on this woman's behalf and want to fight for her against all the injustices she has suffered. That isn't my anger (although I have plenty of my own). It's her anger that I'm feeling, and I'm feeling it because she can't bear to feel it. This is the fury that is expressed in the violence of eating disorders. There is nothing gentle about them; they are not pleasant or nice. They are extremely powerful. Think about the ferocious biting, gulping, chewing, swallowing of a binge; think about the hatred that is expressed in refusing to eat. Many people with eating disorders can easily express their hatred and contempt for themselves; but to suggest that those feelings are really meant for someone else: 'No, no: certainly not. Love and peace, sister'.

So when a woman with a tendency to express her feelings by her eating behaviour is made angry, her anger goes underground and reappears as an attack on herself via food. The process is so customary that it is invisible. She literally swallows her anger. Think of this scenario, which I hear repeatedly. A dance student is in class and is reprimanded for something she is not doing correctly. She feels the comment is harsh or unjust and she struggles to control her tears and to stay in the class. She then goes and buys herself chocolate and eats it quickly. Maybe she then goes into another shop and does the same. As soon as she has done this, maybe even while she's eating the chocolate bar, she's filled with violent rage and hatred of *herself*. So it seems. She doesn't see the connection between what happened in class and her eating behaviour. If she goes home to make herself sick or take laxatives, she doesn't feel that as rage with her teacher either. She is totally convinced that she is not an angry person. She feels that she is pathetic and a victim.

When my clients start to feel angry, I feel like standing on the table and cheering, because I know that that is the beginning of the end for the eating disorder. Women don't need feminists to remind them of the cultural embargo on women's anger, but they do badly need to learn that they can be angry without the sky falling on their heads. Think about what you do when you get angry. Do you even know? And what happened when you got angry when you were growing up? Were you allowed to be angry? Were you ever angry?

Of course, it's not as easy as that. Women don't just need permission to be angry, although that helps. (One girl came to see me, her face blazing with triumph, 'I got angry! I got angry!'). Women are also afraid of what their anger will do; they are afraid of its power. Sometimes it is necessary to find a safe person, and a safe place in which to be angry. One woman I worked with went around being nice to everyone. She thought that if she wasn't nice all the time, then no one would like her. Once she got used to me and able to believe that I would stick with her anyway, she used to practise being angry. It wasn't fun for either of us, and I used to cringe when she slammed the door behind her, but it was very, very necessary. It made her feel much better and loosened the grip of her eating disorder.

EATING YOUR WORRIES AWAY

Lastly there are eating disorders which arise as a response to 'worry'. If a woman puts on weight or loses it, there's a common or garden, everyday, kind of explanation often right at hand, 'Oh, she's been worried.' However a more accurate description might be, 'She was trying not to worry.' Everyone has lots of things to worry about – money, exams, relationships, work, families. Many people lead complicated, successful lives, trying to respond to all sorts of demands. Often a solution to all this pressure is to try to obliterate the worry with food or starvation, rather than to think about what is causing the worry.

There is, that is to say, a positive and creative form of worrying, a necessary and desirable form of worrying – 'worry work'. Of course it is possible to worry in a way that prevents any emotional work being done. We can revolve endlessly and pointlessly in our heads about the things that bother us. This is the kind of worrying that gets us nowhere – the worrying whether the back door is locked, the worry whether the house is tidy enough, the worry about money and paying the bills. We can worry about them without ever really tackling the subject of our worries. But there is another form of worry that is valuable and necessary. If I'm lying in bed worrying whether the back door is locked, then I should get out of bed and look. That kind of worry – of appropriate concern – pushes us into doing what we actually need to do. It is this sort of creative worrying that we can fail to do if we use food to prevent it.

Take a common enough situation – a young woman is due to take an examination in two days time. She's worried about it, but she doesn't let herself worry creatively. Instead she sits down with her books, a packet of biscuits and a cup of coffee. She's so distracted by the biscuits, their smell and the look of them that she can't concentrate. She feels she shouldn't have one, but she does and then she wants more. She eats them, one by one, feeling so guilty that she can't concentrate. She's worrying, in a pointless kind of way, about her examination, but she's also using food to stop herself worrying. If she worked at her worry she would know she needs to revise one set of notes tonight and another set tomorrow night and then she might have a chance of passing her examination. At the moment she thinks she's working but really she's wondering whether she should make herself sick because she's eaten a whole packet of biscuits and if she goes on like this she'll be as fat as a pig.

It can go the other way, of course. A woman is going for an interview and decides that she won't get the job until she's thinner. She's so confused about the difference between 'herself' and her appearance that she is trying to improve her chances of getting the job by being thinner. So then she spends the next ten days worrying about weight and food and size and calories and no time at all thinking about how to present 'herself' at the interview. This is a shame because in order to do well at the interview she needs to spend time to prepare her thoughts and ideas. In fact she needs to work at it, but she doesn't. She stops herself from doing necessary worry work.

This is not by any means an exhaustive list of the crises that people may meet in their lives, but it is enough to illustrate the point. Our eating behaviour may cause us little difficulty except in crisis, and then we can suddenly find ourselves bingeing or starving. If we can permit ourselves to make the link between what is going on in our lives and what we are doing with food, we may not have to resort to such a painful way of coping.

4

On being a woman

It is the thesis of this book that compulsive eating in women is a response to their social position.

Susie Orbach, *Fat is a Feminist Issue*

The associations produced by food, the memories and the history of our experience with food that were discussed in Chapter 2 are, of course, not just the property of women. We all, male and female, have a lifetime of eating to remember. However, eating disorders are, very largely, a women's complaint. Why is that? It has already been suggested that part of the answer may be that women tend to express their distress in ways that hurt themselves rather than turning it out and against other people. However, the question has been answered further by feminist writers and this chapter takes a look at some aspects of their understanding of why women are so tormented by issues of size, of food and of eating.

Morag's initial complaint was not that she had difficulties with food but that she was depressed. When she began to talk about her life it didn't seem very surprising: here was a healthy young woman of 20 living a life of such monotony and boredom that she had every right to be depressed. Morag was a student in her second year at university, surrounded on every side by the attractions and stimulus not only of her studies and the student community, but by the cultural and social riches of London.

Amid this plenty Morag lived a rigid and undeviating routine. She got up at the same time, ate her meals at the same time, studied at the same place in the same library at the same time every day. Weekends caused her great anxiety because the structure of her life was not so rigidly provided by lectures and tutorials, so that she performed her domestic chores such as doing her laundry and cleaning her room in the student hostel with the undeviating regularity with which she attended classes. A tiny indication that there might be another Morag hidden somewhere beneath this mass of rules and regulations was provided by her membership of a church choir. But even this activity was undertaken with the same relentless regularity as the rest of her life.

Morag was also considerably overweight and dressed in a parody of middle-aged fashion. Probably her dress style was modelled on her mother's but in any case it conveyed a woman whose sense of her own possibilities of being physically attractive was very much damaged. In fact she looked a boring frump. Gradually, as we talked, more details emerged of Morag's way of life and of her sadness and despair. She had some female friends at the church she attended, and occasionally went out with them. Similarly she had found another woman at her hostel. The pair of them used to meet each evening at 10 p.m. to drink hot chocolate before bed-time at 10.30. Part of Morag stoutly defended this way of living. She found academic work difficult so she needed lots of time to study – she needed to copy out her lecture notes each day, it was her way of learning. She didn't want to go out in the evenings – it made her too tired the next day. She didn't want to go to parties as crowds of people made her anxious. Besides, sometimes she did go to films with her friends.

But with another part of her Morag was lonely, unhappy and dissatisfied. She was particularly concerned about her weight and size. 'If only' she constantly said, 'if only I was thinner I wouldn't feel so bad. I wouldn't mind going out if I didn't feel as if everyone was looking at me, thinking "God, she's fat".' Gradually she was able to tell me about her struggles with food and how she sometimes spent the weekend in a frenzy of misery.

What was it all about? In time Morag was able to tell me about her family, and then the picture became a little clearer. Her father was a bully and a drunkard who terrorised his wife and two children. He was capable of violent rages especially if some detail of the domestic arrangements failed to please him. Morag's mother was a drudge in this household, afraid of her husband and abused by him. He had many ways of maintaining his tyranny not least of which had been to deprive his family of money. Morag's mother had focused her energies on trying to protect the girls from him.

Not surprisingly, Morag had been glad to escape from this environment and her diligence at school had enabled her to do so via university. However, once there she hardly knew what to do with herself. She had no experience of socialising because she had always been forbidden by her father to go out at night, or to bring friends home. She did not know how to relax and enjoy herself because in order to survive she had created as a schoolgirl a rigid programme of attending to her homework. The undeviating regime she had created at university was her way of continuing this protective system.

But at the same time in some corner of her head Morag knew that there was more to life than the way she was living it. She was curious about boys, but at the same time very frightened of them. In her first year at university she had been invited to the Freshers' Ball, but in total panic had refused the invitation. Since then, however, these anxieties had been overtaken by a constant anxiety about her size. Over and over again she told me that if only she could get thin, her problems would be over.

In due course Morag began to talk about what she might do once she had her degree. She told me that she thought she would like children, but she added she didn't think she wanted a husband, or even a boyfriend. In fact she had wondered if she could make use of the services of a sperm bank. What was it, I wondered aloud to her, that was so unattractive about living with a man. And then out of Morag's mouth came a torrent of words about how horrible men are: how mean, how selfish, how cruel, how unloving. And for a woman to live with a man, I asked? She was a slave, said Morag, taken advantage of, used, a victim. She was much better off on her own.

Morag did not consciously know that she was describing her parents and the relationship between them. Like most of us she assumed that her experience was how it was for everyone. More than most of us, she had had little opportunity for discovering any different. Unconsciously she was convinced that any relationship with a man would place her in the same situation that her mother had been in. Morag's life might be limited but she was not the exploited slave that her mother had become. Her size, her appearance, her way of life, her preoccupation with food were all a way of protecting herself from her mother's fate. She thought of herself as afraid of men and of their sexual impulses, but she was also afraid of her own sexual feelings because they ran the risk of getting her involved with a man.

When Morag began to realise where her image of the role of women came from she began to be able to think about the possibility that there might be other ways of relating to men than the one she saw her mother engaged in. She could begin to think what sort of relationship she might like. As she became less afraid and more hopeful she began to find her problems with food less compulsive and she began to lose weight.

Perhaps Morag represents an extreme example of a woman's rejection of the role of woman presented to her by society. But even if her experience of what it means to be a woman was particularly unpalatable, it provides, I think, a rather good example of how women will use compulsive eating as a protest against being sexual on those terms and as a preoccupation that enables us to push down our sexual feelings. It is very hard to carry on a relationship if you really are absorbed in what you eat, what shape you are and how much you weigh.

THIN IS BEAUTIFUL?

Let us look at this a little more closely. What it suggests is that there is a 'received', accepted shape for a woman to be if she wants to be viewed as a sexual person. This is an idea which has been developed and explored very widely by feminist writers. In particular the link between these pressures and eating disorders has been elaborated in Britain by Susie Orbach and what follows in this chapter owes a lot to her work. If these ideas are meaningful to you for understanding your eating behaviour, then you should certainly read her work, especially *Fat is a Feminist Issue*. (You will find details of this and her other books at the end of the book.)

It is not a particularly new idea that women's shape (or the shape to which women are told they should aspire) is dictated by a force outside women themselves. Hilde Bruch in her work on anorexia named 'fashion' as one of the pressures which urge women towards being thin, and in anorexia gets completely out of hand. Indeed the history of fashion is the history of how different parts of the female body have been emphasised at different times and required to be of a certain size and shape. So, for example, low cut, off-the-shoulder and high-waisted garments have all emphasised the breasts; bustles emphasised the bottom; crinolines emphasised the waist. It is also well known that in the pursuit of fashion women have been willing to do themselves physical harm. The tight, lacing stays to make a woman's waist smaller in the late nineteenth century actually caused distortion of the rib cage:

'Put down that tray and come lace me tighter,' said Scarlett irritably. 'And I'll try to eat a little afterwards. If I ate now I couldn't lace tight enough.' . . .

'Hole onter sumpin' and suck in yo' breaf,' Mammy commanded.

Scarlett obeyed, bracing herself and catching firm hold of one of the bedposts. Mammy pulled and jerked vigorously and, as the tiny circumference of whalebone girdled waist grew smaller, a proud, fond look came into her eyes. . . .

'Now you come eat, honey, but doan eat too fas'. No use havin' it come right back up agin.'

Scarlett obediently sat down before the tray, wondering if she would be able to get any food into her stomach and still have room to breathe.

Margaret Mitchell, *Gone with the Wind*

Our own age is not much different. How many of us have suffered hurt feet and backache from walking or standing in high heels designed to make our feet look dainty and insubstantial? Everybody knows the expression 'Il faut souffrir pour être belle' — you have to suffer to look beautiful. How it translates more accurately is 'a *woman* has to suffer to be beautiful'.

What feminist writers have done, however, is to draw attention to how these ideas about what shape women should be, come from outside us. It is not we individually who decide, for example, that this year it will be trendy to show our knees. Fashion is part of an expectation that women will look the way that society wants them to look. It is true, of course, that in terms of fashion in clothes these changes and requirements are far less absolute than they used to be. In terms of body shape there are continuing changes of emphasis from breasts to waist, to legs, to bottom, but the overriding requirement of these externally imposed visions of women is that they are thin.

Those national models of how to be a woman, the Princess of Wales and the Duchess of York (whom we are encouraged to pretend are just like us when the popular press calls them Di and Fergie) are the subject of endless comment about their weight. Princess Diana became rapidly and visibly thinner after her marriage, and enormous pressure was exerted on the Duchess of York to get her to lose weight. Evidently it is of supreme importance that these two role models get *thin*.

Think for a moment of the images of women presented to us, and the multitude of means of doing so. The advertising industry depicts women on TV, on billboards, in magazines and in newspapers. By these endless visual images we are shown women whose sexual success, attractiveness, wealth, leisure, beauty, youth are all associated with being thin – and of course with whatever product is being promoted.

Now there are very few people who do not wish to be sexually successful, etc, etc. In whatever way they would define those states for themselves, women seem to have bought the message that to achieve these goals they have to be thin. In pursuit of thinness, we spend amazing amounts of money on products which are sold on the basis that they will help keep us thin. Yoghurt, for example, whatever its other merits and food value, is sold very often as a 'slimming food'. Evidently we have been so beguiled by this notion that we need to be told that 'slimming foods' will only aid weight loss as part of a calorie controlled diet. Few women do their food shopping without at the same time thinking of what will or will not keep them thin.

Yet considering all the money and pressure from inside and out, not to mention the time, concern and worry, we seem to make an extraordinarily poor job of keeping thin. It is not necessary to see the actuarial statistics of life assurance companies to know that large numbers of women (and men) are carrying considerably more weight than their frames can manage comfortably, let alone more than the advertising industry decrees. What is more, if we do succeed in getting rid of the extra weight, what do we do but put it straight back on again'? Various studies all point to the same conclusion – that virtually all weight lost is regained within two years. In *The Rotation Diet*, the author, Martin Karahn (Bantam 1987), compares the weight loss success story of his institute in St Louis, Missouri, with that of other groups. In comparisons given to prove the success of the institute's own methods, he indicates that in some weight loss programmes the weight gain after the end of the programme was more rapid than the weight loss during it.

The failure to achieve or maintain weight loss is, of course, put down to lack of persistence, lack of will power, lack of moral fibre, and so on. What feminists have done is to turn this on its head and say that maybe women *don't* want to be thin, that maybe their continuing failure with diets and weight loss, and the way they maintain their fat with compulsive eating, is in some way intentional. Maybe fat serves a purpose for women. And maybe that purpose is to protest against the way women's bodies are objectified and abused, and to protest against the powerless role in society to which women have been relegated.

WOMEN'S POSITION IN SOCIETY

This is not the place to demonstrate point by point the oppression of women, but it is worth just outlining some of the arguments that have been put forward showing how women's place in society is disadvantaged. The economic arguments show first of all that the vast majority of the work that women do in home-making and childcare is unpaid. Since we live in a society where work is valued according to how it is rewarded financially, women's work has come to be regarded as valueless often by the women themselves ('I'm just a housewife') as well as by those around them. Yet whenever the real cost of housekeeping and childcare has to be paid on the open market (housekeepers, nannies, cleaners), the cost of paying for the number of hours a woman works at these tasks is enormous. Secondly when women do work outside the home, their work is less well rewarded, even where they do the equivalent work to men. They do those jobs that have the least status, the fewest prospects of promotion. Proportionately they have far fewer senior positions. They earn less, they inherit less, and therefore in financial terms they control much less. Many, many women have no financial independence from their husbands at all.

The social arguments demonstrate how much of this financial impotence comes about. Women are less well educated, get fewer years of schooling, less training, attend higher and further education in smaller proportions than men, go on to advanced study in smaller numbers. None of this seems to be related to ability or to perceived potential, but to social expectation. There is a wide expectation that after a year or two's work, usually unrelated to a career structure, women will marry and start a family. Their participation in the work world thereafter is anticipated to be part-time and again unrelated to a career structure.

Now it is undeniable that the women's movement has achieved some remarkable changes of attitude and that these inequalities are being eroded. For example, in the mid-sixties roughly one-third of university places in Britain went to women, two-thirds to men. In the mid-eighties almost half go to women. Again, it is still true that women work part time but it is also true that employers are increasingly willing to adapt conditions to women's needs, for instance with regard to holidays and hours. However, there are internalised attitudes in both men and women that prolong oppression and are much harder to erode in either sex.

Parallel to these aspects of women's lives is their sexual oppression. Women's bodies are degraded by their use as sales gimmicks (the model draped across the bonnet of a car), by their depiction in newspapers and magazines, in soft and hard pornography (page 3 of the *Sun,* and many readily available pornographic magazines such as *Playboy, Penthouse, Esquire,* etc). Sexual harassment of women is exceedingly common (wolf-whistles, touching up, flashing) and sexual assault on women inside and outside relationships is not only common, but often not treated as crime ('she brought it upon herself . . . she was asking for it').

If we now return to the story of Morag, it is perhaps easier to see how she had understood her mother's experience and how she wanted no part of it. Her mother was 'just' a housewife, a 'stay-at-home mum', as Morag described her, and totally dependent financially upon her husband. There was not the least pretence of equality in the home – he was the important one, the breadwinner, the head of the household. At the same time he used his position to maltreat his family both physically and emotionally. Is it surprising that Morag recoiled against the lifestyle of her mother? Her compulsive eating was her way of protecting herself against that fate.

FAT AS A MESSAGE

Susie Orbach has done some extremely interesting work with women in which she has been able to get to the positive meanings that women give to their fat. Of course we are all familiar with the routine of hating ourselves because we are fat, feeling loathing and contempt for what we put into our mouths, feeling disgust with our size and shape (however unreasonable all of that may be on any rational understanding). What is much more interesting is to identify what we might be trying to accomplish by our resolute refusal to be thin.

Orbach identifies two major purposes in the behaviour of the compulsive eater. One is power and the defiance of the impotent image of women. The other is anger. A characteristic of the physical images of women most often presented to us by the media is their physical fragility. Women are often shown (and indeed often clothe themselves) in garments that make physical comfort and exertion impossible. It is impossible to run in high heels and a tight skirt. But aside from that, women are shown without any kind of muscle development at all. And of course being thin they do not weigh very much. By this means the ordinary fact that men are usually taller, heavier, stronger, is turned into a gross imbalance. Men are encouraged to physical development, exertion, competition; women are inhibited from it. With that physical fragility is often shown an intellectual incapacity. Some women actually pretend to be stupid in order to maintain an intellectual imbalance to match the physical (pretending not to know how the car works or not even learning to drive; refusing to learn how to operate the computer; not bothering to understand pensions or life assurance). And then with those goes a kind of emotional feebleness – women cry rather than get angry, sulk rather than say what they think.

No wonder a lot of us want to dissociate ourselves from all of this. Some of us manage to do so directly. There are far more models of strong women about – in athletics, in business, in politics – and more of us are managing to assert ourselves as women. But this is often extremely difficult within the social and cultural context in which we find ourselves, and for some of us the attempt remains indirect. The way some of us seem to have found of trying to be powerful is by increasing our bulk, by abolishing in some sort of metaphorical way our fragility, our weakness, our impotence. Valerie was someone who had been sexually abused as a child. From an early age she was sexually active herself. She was a very big woman, tall, strong and heavy. Despite her size (or because of it) she was a considerable athlete and competed on equal terms with men both at squash and tennis. She was fiercely competitive and therefore a challenging opponent at these games. In due course the local male squash champion sought her out to play. Their games were hard fought but usually the man won. Valerie realised that in order to have greater speed around the court she needed to lose some weight. She duly put herself on a diet and began to lose weight. Her competitiveness and perseverance served her as well in this as in her sport. Steadily over the weeks and months she took off her weight and sure enough was speedier around the court and began to win her squash games. Then she stopped. Not because she had got to the weight that she had set herself, but because she began to feel less powerful, less in command, less in control. It was as if her sense of being strong, of having authority, of being someone to reckon with, was identified completely with her size. If she lost too much weight she would be vulnerable and in danger. That fear was, of course, related to her actual experience as a sexually abused child. In her sexual relationships as an adult she had refused to allow herself to be too vulnerable, too drawn in, and with men and women she had used her physical size, weight and strength to make sure she would never if she could help it again join the ranks of the weak and powerless. But with her size she also expressed her fury, which she could not yet feel emotionally, about how she had been exploited. Her size expressed the reality that she was and would be no longer a victim.

Wendy had been married for years and had delayed having a child because of her interest in her work and her developing career. The time came, however, with the biological clock ticking away, when it was time to start having children if that was what she was going to do. In fact she and her husband found it very difficult to conceive. There seemed to be no biological impediment, although various medical authorities told Wendy to lose weight to bring down her blood pressure, but this she seemed to find impossible. She was considerably overweight and had been for years. But one thing was clear to Wendy – just as soon as she did have a baby she would resign from work. In the meantime, however, she found herself another job, more rewarding and more prestigious than she had dreamed possible. She did not, however, lose weight. It began to be clear that all Wendy's anxieties about what she would lose if she had a child were expressed in her size. Perhaps there were also anxieties about what she would gain. She *looked* permanently pregnant, as if to satisfy that part of her that wanted to have a child, but there was a stronger force that made her very reluctant to

give up her power in the world in exchange for motherhood. Yet
she had created for herself such an ideal of motherhood that she
was unable to express that conflict except by her size.

Mrs Yates was the large wife of a clergyman. More even than
most women she was defined by her husband's job. Part of her
role was to be professionally 'nice': kind, good-tempered, despite
however else she might be feeling. Indeed there seemed also to be
a professional embargo on 'feeling' anything but 'nice'. Certainly
Mrs Yates did not know she was anything but nice although an
acute observer might have noticed a fair number of sour comments and disparaging judgments. It was hard for her to see that
she stifled her resentment at the role she had to play, her rage at
the way her own considerable talents had not been allowed to
develop – because of course a woman in her position couldn't go
out to work. Oh no, her husband needed her too much. Even
when directly asked if she did not feel angry at the limitations of
her existence, she would deny it. The only way her anger could be
expressed was by the biting and swallowing of food.

There are two things to be said about compulsive eating as a
way to deal with our dissatisfaction and distress about our social
role as women. The first is that it does not work. In fact it is an
exceedingly painful and difficult way to live. Nobody can enjoy
the craving to eat irrespective of physical need. It is an extremely
painful addiction that has to be carried on in secret and is full of
shame and guilt. Just because a compulsive eater's binge may be
no more than a couple of chocolate bars does not make it any easier. There is something frightening and humiliating about the
desperate need to eat. When it means a binge followed by vomiting and purging, then the compulsive eater finds it hard to hang
on to any shred of self-esteem, let alone what it does to the way
she feels physically. Alice used to come to work looking truly
terrible, her face bloated, her eyes bloodshot, pale as a ghost. In
the beginning her colleagues used to comment and ask her what
was wrong, but her evasive replies and embarrassment soon made

them stop. Alice could only imagine them speculating behind her back on what she did to make herself so ill. This worry made her keep herself apart from her workmates until she was leading an extremely isolated existence.

Not only is it a painful way to live; it also does not begin to deal with the problem. In this chapter we have been considering the idea that compulsive eating may be a response to a woman's perception of her social role. By misusing food a woman may be making a statement about what she feels about her life as a woman. But this issue is not in any way tackled or dealt with by the eating behaviour. In fact it is a way of *not* knowing about or dealing with these issues. It is a translation into eating behaviour of feelings. Those feelings may be any of a large range – fear, anger, envy, despair – but they are feelings that we evidently feel we cannot know about or deal with, that somehow have to be magicked away and make a reappearance as eating behaviour.

It is true, of course, that the feelings *are* hard to deal with. Mrs Yates had been trained for so long and so thoroughly never to know that she had an unkind or an angry thought or feeling that to acknowledge that (like the rest of us) she had a good many such was very, very hard. And also like the rest of us, Mrs Yates was very judgmental about such ideas and feelings. She thought they were bad, wicked, wrong. She was very unaccepting of herself and found it hard to distinguish between a thought or a feeling which has no moral value and an action which may have moral value. So, for example, she found it hard to take in the idea that feeling angry about the way her husband presumed that she would be willing to sacrifice her life and her career for his life and his career might be a very appropriate response. But she *was* angry about it and she showed her anger in ways she did not allow herself to recognise, especially by her eating.

However, there was something else that Mrs Yates found hard to deal with, and also hid from herself with her fat and her pre-occupation with food, and that was the extent to which she had agreed to be her husband's deputy. She would say that of course she hadn't expected to go on working when she married a clergyman and that in fact she had been quite glad to give up work; besides, helping her husband in the parish was very rewarding; there were lots of people in need and it was good to be able to help out. At a deeper level, though, she blamed her husband for stifling her career and her prospects and she was in some ways an embittered and unforgiving woman.

None of that was easy to deal with for Mrs Yates, nor would it be for any of us. What is more, there was no way of putting it right. Unlike Emma, she no longer had her life before her. Her opportunity to develop her career was by this time over; she was an elderly woman. Yet there was a lot to be gained by allowing herself to know about her true feelings. For a start she need no longer spend her days preoccupied with food and thinking about the next meal; but also she had the opportunity to grow and develop as a person, as a woman, as a human being. There was emotional work that desperately needed to be done in Mrs Yates's life. There was need to grieve for what had not happened, for the opportunities missed and the potential unrealised. There was need to achieve a more honest relationship with her husband, to stop sniping at him indirectly and to begin to attempt to be more direct about her own feelings. Most of all there was need for her to consider how she was going to live the last part of her life and how she could use the remaining years as creatively as possible. Compulsive eating was a way of surviving, not of living.

What we have to come to terms with is that we may be unable to right the wrongs of women, in our own case, in our own lifetime. We may also have to accept that we will pay a high price for taking responsibility for our own lives. If your refusal to accept your role leads you to end a relationship, for example, then you do have something very hard to deal with. On the other hand you will at least be living your life, rather than postponing it by compulsive eating.

Mrs Brown is a giant of a woman. She's been getting that way ever since she first was pregnant. She now has three small boys; the eldest is about 7, the youngest about 2. Every day her husband goes out to work in the morning in a thoroughly conventional way, and she in a thoroughly conventional (and increasingly uncommon) way stays at home and looks after the children. She takes the eldest one to school and the middle one to nursery. Then she comes home with the little one and does housework until it's time to collect the middle one from nursery. They have lunch together. Then Mrs Brown clears up a bit while the little one has his nap. After that they go out so that she can get any shopping she needs on the way to pick up the big one from school. After they all get home Mrs Brown makes tea for the children, clears up again and makes some preparation for dinner for herself and her husband. Then it's time to get the children ready for bed. They've had their baths by the time Mr Brown comes back and he reads them their stories and puts them to bed while Mrs Brown finishes dinner for the adults. By the time they've eaten, cleared up, made some preparations for the next day and watched the news on TV, it's time to go to bed. Both of them are really tired so they don't often make love; they just go straight off to sleep, because the youngest child will wake them pretty early in the morning.

Some women might like this way of living. Mrs Brown hates it – not that she knows. She hides her fury, and her guilt at her fury, and her despair behind her enormous size which she maintains by eating all day long. Her chores are punctuated by food. She feels guilty and miserable about the way she looks and the way she eats, and she wonders if it's her size that makes her husband not want to have sex any more. It's true that her fat can actually make it a bit awkward. And besides, she loves her children and her husband and wants to take care of them. She could do with spending some time thinking about her eating behaviour. Couldn't she?

5

The difficulties of
growing up

On 9 January Margaret came from the ward to my room. . . .
She was accompanied by a nurse, and, in spite of looking as
though her skeleton-like body would be broken into pieces by
the weight of the hospital blanket draped round her shoulders,
she walked steadily and unaided. . . . I explained to her that
treatment entailed her telling me any thoughts that came into
her mind so that together we could try to understand why she
was not wanting to eat. . . . She looked a little less pinched and
cold and gradually moved her body so that she was curled up
under her blanket in such a way that a picture of a baby feeding came immediately to my mind. . . . After a pause, in
response to a slight movement in her body, I said I thought that
she wanted to talk to me with her body as she had done to her
mother before she could talk. . . . Up to this stage in her analysis her unconscious conflicts about growing up had been
expressed mainly through her body in such things as gains and
losses of weight.

Tustin, *Autistic Barriers*
(Karnac, 1987, pages 243–5, 255)

Anorexia was the first of the eating disorders to be studied.
Almost from the beginning it was thought that anorexia was to
do with problems of growing up into a woman. Historically
anorexia began at about the age of puberty which made this

recognition easier. Nowadays the age of onset is not nearly so young on average, but it is still often thought that anorexia relates to a woman's difficulty in 'being a woman'.

The most obvious features of anorexia are the delay or prevention of menstruation and the loss of weight. The loss of weight has sometimes been understood as a way of girls getting rid of the secondary sexual characteristics which include breasts and fat round the hips and bottom. When this understanding of weight loss has been put together with an ending of (or a failure to begin) periods, then it has sometimes been suggested that the point of anorexia, its function so far as the girl is concerned, is to keep her in a pre-sexual state both as far as her hormones and therefore her whole physical self is concerned, and also emotionally. It is a way of remaining pre-sexual emotionally. What follows, then, is the idea that the anorexic girl does not want to grow up, and particularly does not want to grow up sexually.

There are a good number of aspects to growing up, as well as sexual development – the capacity to separate from the family of origin, the capacity to be independent and to make decisions. These and other aspects will be discussed later as they relate both to anorexia and to compulsive eating, but this chapter focuses on developing sexuality as a part of growing up and the way in which it can be halted or reversed by anorexia. These ideas are also related to compulsive eating.

The capacity to come to terms with our sexuality is both desirable and a mark of healthy adult development. For the vast majority of human beings the capacity to form a long-term intimate sexual relationship is the basis of adult contentment and creativity. There are, however, a good number of different ways of handling our sexuality – among them the decision not to have sexual relationships at a certain time or perhaps at all. These decisions are perfectly valid, but cause less pain if they can be made from strength and not from fear. The anorexic's or the compulsive eater's rejection of sexuality is from fear, and it is this aspect that is discussed in this chapter.

This is the moment, perhaps, to mention what is sometimes called 'sub-clinical anorexia'. As anorexia has been so much involved with medical care, it has been treated as an illness by doctors who have drawn up lists defining symptoms. This has been useful in separating anorexia from other illnesses with which it has sometimes been confused and has the advantage of giving a way of behaving and a set of symptoms a name. These symptoms include weight phobia, loss of 25 per cent of body weight or more, refusal to eat and lack of periods. However, this defines the illness chiefly for the benefit of other people, rather than for the sufferer who usually knows very well what is wrong with her. It also excludes from consideration large numbers of women whose anorexic behaviour does not go so far, but is nevertheless real enough.

As with compulsive eating my interest in anorexia is in those who are not happy with the way they use food. Anorexia can be defined, in my terms, as using not eating as a way of expressing emotional distress and having a feeling of compulsion about that way of behaving. This compulsion can last a long or a short time. The point of focus is the behaviour and the attitude rather than whether the drive to not eat goes on long enough to produce a certain set of physical results.

However, it is important to bear in mind what is now understood about the psychological effects of starvation. This point is made in *The Anorexia Reference Book*. With significant weight loss, a weight that may vary somewhat according to the build of the woman concerned, the psychological effects of starvation produce ways of thinking that are delusional and obsessive. Unless there has been some weight gain it is made even more difficult to attempt any kind of psychotherapy.

Returning to the story of Anna that was told partly in Chapter 1, Anna's anorexia had been precipitated by three events: her mother's hysterectomy, her best friend's leaving the country, and her own impending departure for college in London at the age of 18. However, her own later understanding of what it was about was a fear that she would not be able to control her adolescent experimentation, that she was in danger of 'going too far' and that she needed to put the brakes on hard. As she described it, she had as a result been standing still for three years.

Let us think a little more closely about in what way she had been 'standing still'. Clearly not in respect of her studies, since she had completed her course satisfactorily. It was in her social and sexual development that she had stood still. Anna was someone who had begun to have sexual relationships quite early. Yet for three years she had had no boyfriends and no sexual relationship. It was these feelings, these impulses and that behaviour that she got rid of by her anorexia. And in her case her self-starvation had been severe enough and prolonged enough to stop her menstruating. She had returned herself symbolically and literally to a prepubertal state where she was not troubled physically by the evidence of her sexual potential. The hormonal changes brought about by weight loss also remove sexual feelings. Even if that were not so, Anna was far too busy computing calories and worrying about what tiny amounts of food she would eat and when and where to be capable of noticing her sexual impulses. So here was a woman whose growing up had been negotiated well enough at puberty but who found it necessary to reverse that process temporarily at a moment of later crisis.

WOMEN'S SEXUALITY

Feminist writers have provided some ways of thinking further about this kind of behaviour. They point to the ways in which girls are taught from a very early age to control and repress their needs and feelings and instead to respond to the needs of others. The everyday evidence for this exists in the double standard of sexual behaviour where sexual experimentation is appropriate for men, but an equal adventurousness in women will get her called a slag or a whore. Think how many times those words appear in graffiti and how there is no equivalent term for a man. Indeed the equivalent for a man is a term of admiration, a 'jack the lad', a stud. Women are educated to care for the needs of others and that is as true of the sexual sphere as of any other. So women are brought up to respond to a man's sexual needs rather than to know their own, to gratify the man by their response, 'faking it' if necessary and not to expect or demand orgasm and sexual satisfaction themselves.

This is all a poor preparation for the possibility that a woman will indeed experience very urgent sexual needs and desires. She may very well, as Anna did, find herself extremely frightened by the intensity of her feelings and become convinced that she is courting disaster. It was difficult for Anna to accept her feelings and recognise them as ordinary. Perhaps a further element of this difficulty lay in the possibility of her sister's envy. Anna's sister was older, but much less confident and successful socially. It was hard for Anna to accept her own enjoyment and her own feelings when they were not shared by her sister.

Anna's experience of anorexia was bad enough, but she recovered in a fairly short time and had the advantage of having a history of being an adolescent to fall back on. She had well developed social skills; she was accustomed to going out with friends both in groups and with one other person; she had a fairly large circle of acquaintances both male and female; she had been out with boys and she had had some sexual experience. As well as that, she had had a lot of practice in experimenting with and creating an image for herself with clothes and make-up. When she got better she was able to resume where she had left off. It is much more difficult if a girl has never negotiated puberty at all. If a woman puts the brakes on her development then she loses the opportunities of development that Anna had enjoyed. Her fear of growing and development is so intense that it will not allow her even to embark on the journey towards womanhood.

A PSYCHOANALYTICAL APPROACH

One of the ideas psychoanalytic thinkers have had about anorexic girls who seem to have difficulty negotiating puberty and growing up, is that for some of them growing out of being their father's daughter is too difficult.

A young woman from an exceedingly prosperous and comfortable family had a very successful father. He was a distinguished architect and an attractive and charming man. Nancy was his adored daughter. She was pretty, clever, everything her father could wish, and he was extremely proud of her. The pair had a very close, even intimate relationship, which at times excluded Nancy's mother. Nancy would spend whole evenings with her father in his study. They would talk and laugh and sometimes Nancy would sit on his knee. Only two things spoiled this idyllic pleasure. One was that Nancy's father could not bear her to go out with boys. Whenever a boy wanted to date her and came to the house, Nancy's father would make disparaging comments so Nancy very soon felt the boy was no good after all. The other problem was that over the course of her adolescence Nancy had become steadily more anorexic. By 18 she had become bulimic and her life had focused on her eating disorder.

It is not very difficult to see what was going on in this family. In some sense Nancy had become her father's girlfriend (although there was no suggestion whatever of an overt sexual relationship between them). This had been achieved, at least in Nancy's eyes, at the expense of her mother. So you might say that in the competition for her father and his interest and attention, Nancy had won. Moreover, her father had played an energetic role in creating this situation. He had colluded in excluding Nancy's mother and he had also excluded male rivals from the scene by in effect getting rid of any potential boyfriend for Nancy. The results were, however, disastrous for the father's marriage and for Nancy.

Nancy in a way had got what she wanted – the exclusive attention of her father – but she had paid a very high price for it; her whole adolescent development had come to a halt and her conflict had become expressed in a serious eating disorder. She had managed to hold on to her childhood role of 'Daddy's girl', but only by sacrificing her healthy development into a woman. The pair of them were locked into a relationship that was not only long-time expired, but also very destructive.

Some therapists working with anorexics have used methods of family therapy to help not only the sufferer but her whole family. Often it looks as though the meaning of a girl's reluctance to grow up is best understood in terms of the whole family's functioning. Certainly that seems likely in the case of Nancy's family. (Some details of books on families and anorexia are given at the end of the book.)

Anna and Nancy are examples of women who found the transition to adult womanhood extremely difficult. It was not clear to them at the time and indeed, if it had been, there would have been less need for their anorexia. It was their belief that the feelings surrounding sexuality and adolescent development were unmanageable that forced their anorexia upon them. The refusal, however, can take the form of weight gain, rather than weight loss. Compulsive eating can delay the social and emotional development of an adolescent just as effectively as anorexia, although not in such a life-threatening way. However, perhaps in terms of peer group rejection, fat teenagers have a worse time than anorexics. Fat children are tormented by other children and fat teenagers endure torture quite as bad if slightly more subtle. Not long ago I watched a group of American teenagers on a tube in London. They were standing by the door and quite a lot of friendly and flirtatious banter was going on between them. There were several boys and several girls. Among the girls was one who was extremely fat. It was very interesting to see that she was excluded from the pushing and nudging that was going on, and also that comments addressed to her were not personal but factual: 'Where do we change tubes?' rather than the teasing 'What makes you think I want to go out with you?' The fat girl evidently had created the position of tour guide for herself which gave her a place within the group, but she was excluded from the game of 'boy meets girl' which was the reason for the group's existence.

The transition from child to adolescent to adult is not easy and if a girl feels quite inadequate to its challenge she can refuse to negotiate it altogether. At a less desperate level, it is quite probable that we can refuse to negotiate such changes many times in our lives. It is not true that at puberty or in late adolescence we deal with the problems that our developing sexuality presents us with once and for all. On the contrary, we are repeatedly working through these challenges, certainly for the first half of our lives. If we get too frightened, too overwhelmed, our response can be a retreat into eating disorders. An anorexic episode or a binge may last days, weeks or months, and it is none the less real for its shorter duration.

DAISY'S STORY

Daisy was someone who had been anorexic in her mid-teens. She had one brother two years older. Her parents had had a struggle to make a living and in the process the children had suffered some emotional neglect. Probably as a result of this the two children had sought comfort from each other and there had been for some years while they were both prepubertal a physical relationship between them.

This had caused Daisy a very difficult mixture of feelings of pleasure and guilt. This in itself would have made puberty difficult, but Daisy had two further complications to deal with. One was that she was an independent and tomboyish girl who was not very successful at making friends with her own sex, and preferred the company of boys. This tomboyishness is something that feminists have helped us to understand as the reaction of an energetic and lively girl to the limitations of the role of girl that has been presented to her. What is more, the class expectations of Daisy as an adolescent were that she would leave school, marry young and begin to have children soon thereafter. The model of the life that awaited her, as her mother's daughter, was a life of domesticity and of isolation while her husband went out to work. Daisy's father had a business which he greatly enjoyed running, more evidently than he enjoyed being at home with his wife and family, since as a child Daisy saw little of her father. At the same time she saw her mother as weak, passive and devalued, but also vulnerable. When Daisy's parents quarrelled, the quarrels, in Daisy's perception, were always brought to an end by her father saying to her mother, 'Well, if you don't like it, you know what you can do. You can pack your bags.'

So, then, there was difficult early sexual experience for Daisy to deal with. There was a social role that for her was uninviting for a number of reasons, but there was also something else. The father of one of Daisy's friends had exposed himself to her and had showed her pornographic magazines. This had been frightening to Daisy, then about 12 or 13 years old; so frightening and so guilt-provoking was it that she had told no one. She felt herself in some way to blame. All of this she might still have coped with, and indeed did for a while, in that she began to menstruate and to be interested in boys. However, at 15, she was seduced by a much older man. This finally was more than she could deal with and she became anorexic.

What had happened was that Daisy had grown up in an environment where having sexual wishes and feelings carried excitement but also too much guilt and fear. As she got older and those wishes and feelings got stronger, her fear and guilt were not resolved but instead increased to the point where they were simply unmanageable. She got rid of her feelings, her wishes, her sexuality, even her memories for a time, in the wholehearted pursuit of emaciation. She had felt there was no one who could help her deal with her sexuality, no one she could talk to about her fears and her guilt. Now that she was anorexic she made absolutely sure that she did get the attention she needed.

However of course it was the wrong kind of attention. Instead of the understanding and the holding that she needed, she provoked irritation and anger. She came from a family with very conventional eating behaviour. They were a meat and two veg. sort of family for whom Sunday dinner was an important social occasion. Daisy's wish to be a vegetarian, her refusal to eat what her mother cooked, her sitting not eating and not contributing at family mealtimes – all of it provoked concern and then anger, and then despair. Daisy, of course, had no idea what the problem was. I say 'of course' because if she had been able to know what it was that was bothering her, she might not have needed to be anorexic. Her anorexia was about a desperate fear of knowing, a refusal to know. The understanding of what was going on with her that has been described here only came ten years later. She did have sexual wishes, feelings and desires but her belief (and a belief that had a sound basis in her experience) was that such wishes and feelings were too difficult and too painful. She used the anorexia to abolish them.

Despite all this Daisy had not quite given up. She chose a kind, gentle, patient man, a good number of years older than she was herself, and attempted to use the relationship with him to cure herself. The trouble was that she was not only afraid of his sexual needs, his sexuality, she was also frightened of her own. No matter how gentle her lover was it did little for Daisy's fear of her own feelings and sexual capacities. Inevitably the relationship came to an end.

Then even more difficult times began because Daisy had begun to lose the ability simply to go on starving herself and began to maintain her low weight by bingeing and vomiting or purging. The control that Daisy had managed to maintain up to that point was broken and the whole of her life began to be as chaotic as her new eating behaviour. Her sexual appetite, as if to convince her that all of her fears about herself were true, became frantic and desperate. At the same time the bit of her that was still a terrified child was visible from time to time when she became afraid to be left alone in her boyfriend's flat.

In all of this horror there were two points of stability. One was Daisy's parents. Despite their anger and their incomprehension, they had held on. They maintained contact with her; they allowed her to come home whenever she wanted to despite the fact that such visits were often very uncomfortable for everyone. In fact they loved their daughter as well as they knew how. The second point of consistency was Daisy's dancing. During all the painful years of her adolescence and early twenties she was training as a dancer and then teaching dance, both choreography and performance. It would not be true to say that this had been easy. There had been many moments of anguish and despair, but at the same time dancing gave Daisy some self-respect. At least she was working and that helped her to hold on to some sense of her own value.

Very slowly she began to get better. She found herself some therapy and courageously began to look at what had been going on with her. Her eating difficulties did not go away at once or easily. It seemed as though when Daisy felt again the old despair and distress about her sexuality, she would then retreat into her eating disorders for a day or a few days or a week. For example, after a long time of feeling that she would never find a relationship within which she could love and be loved, and within which her sexual needs could be satisfied without hurt or humiliation, she was contacted by a man she had known some years previously. Daisy spent two weeks with him and both of them worked hard on talking about what had happened last time in their relationship and why it had come to an end, and whether this time round

there was something for both of them in being together. Daisy
was initially very cautious and suspicious but gradually relaxed.
It seemed as though the relationship might have a future. The
man left and then within a very short time he stopped telephon-
ing or writing. He did not reply to Daisy's letters and when she
tried to telephone he could not be contacted.

This very brutal rejection would have been painful for anyone,
but for Daisy it seemed to confirm everything she feared. If she
allowed herself to be sexual then the result would be disastrous.
Her response was to retreat into her eating disorder. By that
means she could feel nothing, want nothing, need nothing. The
grieving, the anger, the disappointment, the depression that were
appropriate to this loss were all hidden behind a preoccupation
with food and with weight. But Daisy had in fact learned a great
deal and it was not all that long before she was able to deal with
her feelings more directly and even believe that she was not wrong
or bad for wanting a sexual relationship with this man.

One of the ways of keeping an eating disorder at hand, ready
for such emotional crises, is to belong to a profession where thinness is required. We have already seen in Chapter 1 how Janet
French said that her anorexia/ thinness was because of her dancing and for her dancing, but that eventually it stopped her
dancing because she could no longer control it. There are many
dancers with eating disorders and they live in a culture where
close attention to weight and shape is the norm. In a way this
gives permission for food misusers to continue with their obsessive behaviour. The same could be said of a number of other ways
of life – that of a model, for example, or a gymnast. In each of
these activities there is a high value placed on extreme thinness
and a prepubertal unwomanly shape. They are also environments
which seem to confirm the very unrealistic ideas of body shape
and size that many anorexics have. The criteria for what is and
what is not fat are so unlike the judgments of those issues in the
general population that they permit anxiety over what to every-

one else seems a perfectly slim body. Dancing in particular and the dance world have often been accused of creating anorexia, but perhaps the influence is in fact the other way round – that people who feel as if at any moment they might need their eating disorder gravitate towards an environment where their obsessiveness is less noticeable, more permitted.

There are, however, many of us who from time to time retreat into anorexic episodes, in relation to our difficulties with our sexuality, without necessarily belonging to a culture which has thinness as one of its values. Difficulties in our relationships, or even the prospect of a relationship (and therefore of sexual feelings and needs) can trigger off these times. It is as though we have found for ourselves a hiding place, a retreat, a ritual way of coping, a way of managing our conflicts. Unhappily, of course, these methods do not work – first because they cause us a great deal of pain. The anguish of starving, or of bingeing and starving, is a hard way to deal with difficulties. But secondly these ways of coping do nothing to help us deal with our underlying difficulties. They keep us stuck, fixed, at the same place in our development. They keep us from growing as people. We all have, and we all need, ways of coping, but to try and deal with the painfulness of being a woman by torturing and hurting our bodies must surely be something we need to leave behind.

At least I'll control what I put in my mouth

An image came to her, that she was like a sparrow in a golden cage, too plain and simple for the luxuries of her home, but also deprived of the freedom of doing what she truly wanted to do. Until then she had spoken only about the superior features of her background; now she began to speak about the ordeal, the restrictions and obligations of growing up in a wealthy home.
Hilde Bruch, *The Golden Cage*

Over the past 15 years or so, beginning with the work of Hilde Bruch, but continuing in the work of feminist writers on eating disorders, it has been becoming clear that there is a kind of family and early experience which tends to produce anorexic youngsters – girls and boys, but mostly girls. The anorexia then needs to be understood as a way of responding to that family background.

Before looking at these families and these anorexics in more detail, it is worth repeating some of the general points on which this book is based. First among these is that eating disorders cannot be accounted for by any *one* overarching theory. It is true that some anorexics come from this kind of background and if you are reading this trying to think about and understand your own eating disorders, this particular account may be useful to you – but again it may not. Perhaps you will have to read further and think more about your particular experience. Secondly, although it is anorexia that is being discussed and the examples are mostly of people quite severely affected, the central concern is not so much with whether the illness had been clinically diagnosed, as with the underlying 'anorexic' attitude. Thirdly, although it is anorexia that is talked about, in terms of solutions to the difficulties under consideration, it is not much different from compulsive eating. There are differences – obviously it has some significance why some women refuse to eat and others misuse food in different ways. Nevertheless eating disorders of whatever kind are a variation on the central theme of women using food, weight and shape as a means of expressing their emotional distress.

ROSEMARY'S STORY

There is a kind of family, usually white, usually prosperous middle class, which is intensely protective of its children, especially its girl children. Let me describe such a family. The girl, Rosemary, is five years older than her brother. Her mother doesn't work outside the home. Her father is a successful film producer. His work is very demanding and keeps him away from home a lot. His wife, Rosemary's mother, is lonely and devotes a great deal of time to Rosemary. She has decided that Rosemary will be a dancer and has even chosen which stage school she will go to. She herself would have liked to have become a dancer but it wasn't possible, so she thinks it would be nice if Rosemary could be one. She takes Rosemary to classes and spends a lot of time fixing her hair and her costumes and going with her to dancing competitions. She's very proud of Rosemary's talent as a dancer and is determined that it will be developed. Rosemary is also a very pretty little girl and her mother makes sure that she is always beautifully turned out. Even though Rosemary is now 9 or 10 her mother still chooses what she should wear every day. Rosemary doesn't seem to mind this. In fact she doesn't seem to mind anything. She's quite happy to sit and keep her mother company when she gets home from school. She's a very good little girl. In fact in comparison to other girls of her age she's abnormally good. She doesn't seem to want to go to her friends' houses to play and they don't get invited to her house. Rosemary likes her mother's company best and her mother takes her everywhere she goes. Of course Rosemary has to be good when she goes out with her mother.

Rosemary's mother, as will be obvious from this account, was herself very needy, and used her daughter as her companion and friend. She could not allow Rosemary the kind of independence that she desperately needed if she was to grow up capable of living a separate existence. There are plenty of mother-daughter relationships like this that continue throughout the lifetime of both parties and are repeated in the next generation. These are the sorts of relationships where mother and daughter consult each other compulsively on every aspect of their lives, where the relationship between mother and daughter has to take precedence over any other relationship.

Often in such situations it is hard, if not impossible, for the daughter to do something that she knows her mother would not like. Rosemary knew very well that her mother wanted her to be a dancer. Through a whole series of circumstances, including the fact that she became too tall to be a ballet dancer, that did not happen. Rosemary's mother has since died, but Rosemary, now in her mid-twenties, has no idea what she might do instead. In fact so impossible did it seem for her to do anything else, to defy her mother as it seemed to her, that she could not begin to think about what she wanted to do. It was as if she had never learned to want, except to want what her mother wanted for her.

FELICITY'S STORY

Now Rosemary's family is the kind of family that can produce an anorexic. Let's think about Felicity and her family. Felicity is in her late teens and very, very thin. She has an exceedingly slender and fragile neck which makes her look very frail and vulnerable. She comes from a family where her father is a successful businessman.

She has one sister who is two years older and a mother who, as long as Felicity can remember, has stayed at home and spent all her time and energy on looking after her family. They have a lovely new house and it is beautifully clean and well looked after. Since she was born Felicity has been taken care of very well. She has always been able to have pretty much what she wants materially – in fact it has been her parents' pleasure to provide it for her. Nowadays she has some nice clothes, much nicer than most of her contemporaries, but she looks after them much more carefully than they do theirs anyway, and makes sure that they are clean and ironed. Her mother does most of that for her.

One of the ways in which Felicity's mother has tried to take the best possible care of her is in providing food. When Felicity was a schoolgirl her mother was always there in the afternoon when she got home from school with something to eat to carry her over till dinnertime. Whenever she goes anywhere her mother provides her with a beautifully thought out and put together packed lunch, and nowadays whenever she gets home from work there is a meal waiting for her.

This business of food is difficult for Felicity and has been for quite a long time. When she was a schoolgirl she used sometimes to tell her mother that she didn't need to be there every day; she, Felicity, was old enough to take care of herself; wasn't there something that her mother wanted to do for herself? But her mother said no, she didn't mind being there when Felicity came home, and anyway, she felt it was her duty. She wouldn't feel at all easy about Felicity coming home to an empty house.

Over the last few years Felicity has become very thin indeed, partly because she turns down a lot of what her mother offers her. Of course this makes her mother very anxious and she presses food on Felicity, but that only makes her even more determined not to accept it. She feels that her mother wants her to eat more than she should. In any case, these days Felicity does a lot of dancing and needs to be thin to go on with that.

It seems clear that Felicity is using food and her capacity to refuse to eat her mother's food as a way of trying to separate herself from an intensely close, concerned and protective family. Her big sister is a bit tougher than Felicity in some ways. When she was growing up she had rows and disagreements with her parents. This won for her sister her freedom and independence so that she has now gone off to university in another city and has created a life and a circle of friends of her own. Felicity was frightened by these rows and saw how much they upset her parents. Besides she feels she was never allowed to get angry or to answer back and she doesn't really know how to defy them.

This is not to say that Felicity hasn't tried to strike out a bit on her own. She has, but it is difficult because her parents want to do everything for her, and when she does try and do something for herself it never seems to work out, or at least never as well as when her parents do it for her. Take for instance the first time she decided to move out of home and get a place for herself. She was determined to do it on her own. She looked in the newspapers and tried to team up with other people to get a place, but it kept falling through. Finally she decided to go it on her own and use a flat agency. The agency found her a flat and charged her a huge fee. However, the flat was really pretty horrible, dirty and not in a very good part of town. Within a few weeks Felicity decided it really wouldn't do. This incident left Felicity with a tremendous sense of failure. When she had summoned up all her courage (and it had taken a lot) to try and move out of home, she had made a mess of it.

It makes it more complicated that with part of her Felicity doesn't in the least want to separate from her parents. In some ways their endless concern is irritating. She wishes they wouldn't phone her every day, or at least wait for her to phone them. But on the other hand her own home is beautifully clean, whereas the shared areas of the flat where she now lives are dirty. Besides everything is so convenient and so ready to hand in her parents' home.

When she doesn't know what she really wants in all these other areas Felicity finds some comfort in at least taking control over what she puts into her mouth. She is very health conscious, and a vegetarian, and there are many things she would not dream of eating. When so much of the rest of her life feels unsatisfactory, Felicity can at least create one corner where it feels as if she is in charge.

But she is not very much in charge even in this corner, as she knows all too well. She doesn't know when she's hungry or what she wants to eat, or how much is a good amount to eat any more than she knows what she wants in other directions. She has had very little practice in knowing what she wants – even whether she wants juice or milk, or a whole or a half glass. Her mother made those choices and decisions. But she has had a lot of practice in knowing what other people think she should have. As far as the anorexia goes, she has made up a lot of rules about what she will and won't eat, and that makes her feel more as if she knows what she wants. But of course it's a very difficult system to maintain, and it takes up a lot of energy.

As far as Felicity is concerned, her anorexic behaviour seems to symbolise two things. One is her conflict about whether she does or doesn't want to try and be separate from those parents of hers. Of course practically speaking while she is so thin there is no way that they are going to relax their hold. They don't think she looks after herself properly and they are right, although they have no real idea of how badly she does. This holding on that she has ensured will continue symbolises the side of her that finds the idea of separation utterly terrifying and feels that 'living her own life' is something she is quite incapable of doing.

The other part of the story, though, is the way that Felicity feels that her life depends on the degree to which she can hold her mother's smothering love at arm's length. When she rejects her mother's food (and then the food her own internal mother tempts her to eat) she is rejecting a love that feels to her as if it traps her in a state of permanent dependency. With part of her she wants above all else not to be dependent. Dependency feels infinitely dangerous. She is denying her need for food/love, keeping it out.

If Felicity wanted either of these things alone – dependence or independence – things would be much simpler. But she has tremendous conflict inside her, not only in her body. If we remember what feminists have been saying we might also add that Felicity's mother is perhaps not a very encouraging model for Felicity. Her mother is practically and emotionally totally dependent on Felicity's father, yet within that dependency her function is to look after everybody else; that is what her life is about. How does Felicity dare to grow up and be separate? How does she dare not to?

But remember, fortunately Felicity's older sister has managed these difficulties rather well and her example is intensely important. Slowly Felicity begins to be able to feel and to voice some of her conflicts and, in the process, her eating problems. It involves a change for her parents, too, because they have to learn how to let their child grow up and therefore how to see themselves differently. Felicity's mother particularly has invested a great deal in her mothering. Can she find a way of developing herself now that her children are grown up and will her husband also be able to adjust to the changes in his wife's role, as well as in his own? They both find it painful that Felicity now struggles to express to them the ways in which she feels they have failed her. They did love her, and they do love her, and they did what they did with the best will in the world.

There are lots of hopeful features about Felicity's life, not the least the fact that her anorexia has never taken over her life the way it can do. She works and she has been able to let herself know enough about her mixed feelings about growing up, about separation and independence, above all about her mother, so that she has not had to express everything through her body. As she can feel and explore these difficult areas more there is a very good chance that she will be able to make a complete recovery.

ELISABETH'S STORY

In a way Felicity's situation and her way of dealing with it is fairly easy to understand. Elisabeth's is much more complicated. She too comes from a prosperous, conventional, middle-class household. Her father, like Felicity's, began with very little, has worked hard for his success, and has been proud of his ability to provide generously for the material needs of his wife and two children, Elisabeth and a boy, two years older. Her mother now works as a teacher, but for a lot of her children's childhood she stayed at home because she wanted to provide a secure home for them. She has been intensely protective of Elisabeth who remembers her childhood as a time of never being allowed to do anything for herself, or on her own.

Until puberty all went reasonably well, although Elisabeth now thinks that her mother's anxieties about what 'other people' would think made spontaneity and freedom in behaviour and relationships very difficult. But when Elisabeth reached puberty she began to be intensely pressured by the expectations of her parents. Her mother was apparently afraid of Elisabeth's approaching womanhood and did her best to deny its existence. For example, she would not allow Elisabeth to buy a brassière when Elisabeth wanted and felt she needed to. She herself had only ever had one boyfriend, Elisabeth's father, whom she had met at 16, fallen in love with and married some years later. This model was held up to Elisabeth as the one that was desirable. Her daughter's wishes to explore and experiment with friendships with boys was met with fear and resistance. At the same time Elisabeth's father had strong academic ambitions for his daughter. He wanted her to go to Oxford (as he himself had not done) and felt that a social life was simply a distraction from this more serious aim.

It took Elisabeth until she was 17 to assert herself in the face of these parental expectations. But at that point she insisted on having more of a social life and at the same time continued with her studying for A Levels. Still, looking back at it, she feels that even then there were signs that she was dealing with her difficulties by the use of food. She remembers that she was unable to study unless she was at the same time eating sweets, very little else. Thinking about the insights that feminist writers have given us, perhaps we can understand this sweet eating as a way of dealing with her anxiety about whether her academic and social ambitions could be reconciled: can clever girls be sexy? Marilyn Lawrence has written recently about the way that 'education' can pose hideous problems for clever girls who have grown up in a world where many men are threatened by clever, educated women. Evidently men still marry women younger and less educated than themselves. It is easy to see what kind of a tight corner Elisabeth might be getting herself into, and how hard it was likely to be for her to know what she wanted for herself.

Still, she was managing not too badly and might have survived these conflicts without too much anguish, but sadly she had one pressure too many to deal with. She had left school and won a place at a university – not Oxford – when her boyfriend was killed in a car accident. This was doubly traumatic for Elisabeth since after a series of relationships in which she had been careful not to get too involved, she had allowed herself to become very dependent on this particular young man. Her first year at university was a year of anorexia which resulted in her dropping out.

In some ways Elisabeth's anorexia had much in common with Felicity's. Like Felicity, Elisabeth's anorexia expressed both her anguish about dependency and her need to reject the stifling kind of love that her parents seemed to offer, instead to take control of her life, but at the same time showing to all the world by her thinness her desperate need of care and concern. Elisabeth had conformed to her father's wish that she should go to university, while at the same time knowing in some corner of her mind that it was not for her. Yet it was impossible for her to confront and oppose her father. Her anorexia was in part a translation into physical terms of her need to defy him. Of course she did not know that. If she had known it she might not have needed to do it. Her anorexia achieved the desired result very effectively – she dropped out of university. By the time she decided on a different path to follow, her father was so anxious about her that he was glad to go along with whatever Elisabeth wanted to do.

However, Elisabeth's anorexia was more complex than that. In part it was to assert some control over her life by defying her father, but it was also to deny and keep at arm's length the sexual and emotional needs that had allowed her to make a relationship with a man in which she was dependent. Her dependency as a child had resulted in the stunting of her necessary and ordinary development towards independence and separation. She both craved and was terrified of her dependency needs. When she finally permitted herself to experience dependency with a boy, he was then killed. What Elisabeth learned from this was once again that dependency was too dangerous. Her anorexia said 'I have no needs', but her body shape said 'My needs are not being met.'

To summarise briefly, there appears to be a sort of family which stifles the growth towards independence and separation of its girl children (and more rarely its boys) by over-protectiveness, by intrusiveness, by not allowing those daughters enough room to develop. Sometimes those girls will rebel against that state of affairs by anorexia. In these cases anorexics can be seen both as rejecting what will otherwise stifle, and as a way of taking control of a little part of their lives (but in the end all of their lives). In some ways anorexia is a deafening 'NO', shouted by someone who has never learned to speak.

THE SILENT SIGNALS

It is this 'NO' that is the most obvious part of the illness. Anyone who has ever dealt with anorexics can testify to what a deafening shout it is, and how powerful it is in getting other people to co-operate and obey. It is so frustrating and frightening for other people that it can provoke reactions just as violent. Perhaps that is why people treating anorexics are quite often cruel. The massive rejection is not easy to bear.

However it is very important to remember that the message given by the anorexic is after all *not* that clear. We must also remember that this scream 'NO' is not the only message that an anorexic is giving (or that we are giving in our anorexic episodes). What must not be forgotten is that weight loss and not eating are also both public statements of something very different: of need, of dependency, of fragility. The problem for an anorexic, or indeed for anyone with eating disorders, is that she is caught in a very tight corner. With one part of us we want one thing and want it desperately, but with another we want something quite different, and want that with equal passion. The struggle, the battle, gets fought out for those of us with eating disorders, over food.

The 'NO' of the anorexic produces responses in other people which activate their 'yes'. As has already been noted, many anorexics belong to the 'thin' professions such as dancer, model, gymnast. One of the interesting features of those ways of life for thinking about anorexia is that they demand that a woman's body is on show. Weight loss will quite certainly be noticed in this context, and even very moderate weight loss of a few pounds. In other words an anorexic in these environments is making absolutely certain that she will be noticed. Now if her 'no' were simply 'no', then there is no way that she would want to display her body. Of course it is also true that anorexics bundle themselves up in lots of clothes, deny that they are thin and so on, but it is a very readily noticeable symptom. In other words, it seems as if they want other people to see and to know about their anorexia (and simultaneously don't want them to). And why is that? Because they need other people to say 'yes' for them. Sometimes the 'yes' of other people ('I want you to eat something; you're not eating enough; you're getting terribly thin; I'm worried about you not eating') is used in part by an anorexic as a way of holding on to her 'NO' (if you say 'yes' I'll say 'NO') and becomes part of the meaning of the anorexia. The struggle between yes and no becomes part of the struggle for power, for control, in a woman's life. However, even quite short-lived and sub-clinical anorexia is also very frightening, as well as being exciting and defiant. The anorexic needs to know that even if she will not for the moment say 'yes', there are other people who will say 'yes' for her.

In the end, of course, no one can say 'yes' for us if we will not find the 'yes' in ourselves. Doctors, hospitals, parents will go to all sorts of extreme lengths to say 'yes' for us – forced feeding, intravenous drips, behavioural programming, and so on. However, we all have the power to say 'no' to life, to love, to food. If in the end we decide that this 'NO' is all we can say, then we can do that; we can die, as so sadly some women do, or as tragically we can destroy our lives with a constant preoccupation with food, weight, size. This life, this now, is all we have. It seems so sad to throw it away.

Fortunately, however, there are comparatively few anorexics who are so desperate. What many do instead is to fight out that yes and no in their bodies, using food to do it with – which is exactly what happened with Elisabeth. She had a year of what might be called straightforward anorexia. She didn't eat very much and what she ate she consumed secretly and on her own. She lost a great deal of weight and became a recluse, holed up in her room in a university hall of residence, not working, not going to classes. Finally someone noticed and intervened. She was found medical and psychological help and in the course of about six months made at least a partial recovery.

So far, so good. Elisabeth's anorexia had actually been quite effective in some ways. Her fight to control her life had in some areas been won – she was out of university and exploring other educational possibilities. However this was only one element of Elisabeth's anorexia. Her eating disorder was also a response to her boyfriend's death and was to do with her difficulties with dependency and intimacy. Her anorexia was then partly to do

with a rejection of these things, and therefore also a rejection of sexuality. Compared to the complexity and painfulness of all this, her victory over her father was not very much. She had abolished her dependency needs; she had said a resounding 'NO' to intimacy, but that left her isolated and with very painful needs for someone else. After all, you will remember that Elisabeth had been brought up in a family where there had been very little opportunity for her development as a separate, independent human being. With part of her she was terrified by her isolation and found it difficult and painful being on her own.

In a person without the need to translate these conflicts into eating behaviour they might have emerged in the form of a series of intense relationships, made and broken off – a pattern of can't do with it, can't do without it. In fact what Elisabeth did was enter into an exceedingly dependent relationship with a man, but a man who had himself had very difficult and deprived beginnings and was himself struggling with his dependency needs. He could not meet her needs in any very creative way because he had the same difficulties to confront. So Elisabeth found herself addicted to someone who couldn't really help her, but who needed her desperately and so constantly reinforced her dependency on him.

Elisabeth did not analyse any of this then. She couldn't. So far as she knew she was desperately in love. Then she began vomiting up her food. It was as if she enacted with her body what she could not recognise in her relationship. She needed and wanted closeness, sex, intimacy. More than that, with a bit of her she wanted to be a baby, a tiny child, looked after every minute of the day, attended to in every tiny detail, never left alone, held and cuddled and caressed and protected. So she wanted to eat, to take in, to be nourished, fed, sustained by good food. But at the same time she wanted to be her own woman, dependent on no one, alone, on her own, doing her own thing, not stifled by someone else's presence. Closeness, sex, another person's demands on her produced rage and hate and panic. So she got rid of what she had put inside her.

She forced out of her body those good things that she had just put inside it. They had become bad, poisoning, hurtful to her. Not that she said that to herself. What she said was that she had eaten too much and that she was a greedy pig and would get fat and ugly, so she had better get rid of it.

It is clear that so far as food was concerned Elisabeth was operating in terms of all or nothing. Either she binged or she starved, feasted or fasted. If she ate anything she would eat too much. Yet this had its emotional aspect too. Either she was totally independent, isolated, without relationships, or she was engulfed, smothered. Either extreme had its good points and its bad. The ferocity of the conflict produced her bulimia, the violent and rapid swing between 'yes' and 'no'.

There could be no resolution to this horrible dilemma until Elisabeth could believe that there was more possible in relationships than these violent extremes. Gradually she began to talk to her parents and to express some of what she felt about the past. Slowly the three of them began to work out a way of relating in which Elisabeth no longer treated them either as the enemy or as a bottomless well of resources on which she could draw as she liked. In their turn they began to recognise that their daughter was no longer a child, but a capable and talented young woman with the ability to make decisions about her life. This modification was a great relief to both sides.

This exploration of the alternatives to the extremes of 'yes' and 'no' continued as Elisabeth found a grandmother figure with whom she could discover that there could be care and concern without stifling, and a boyfriend who had sorted out some of his dependency needs and knew how to be separate without being rejecting and how to be intimate without being smothering. And as all this went on Elisabeth's eating disorder began to be less tormenting, less preoccupying. Gradually she began to need that way of expressing herself much less often. The omens for her recovery and development look reasonably good.

7

Mothers and daughters

We are a generation who, with every act of self-assertion as women, with every movement into self-development and fulfilment, call into question the values by which our mothers have tried to live.

Kim Chernin, *The Hungry Self*

Over the past 50 years those who are concerned with the effect early experience has on later life have increasingly turned to look at the part the mother has played, and away from the role of the father. This has not always had very creative results. Fathers and their influence have been ignored while at the same time 'bad' mothers have been blamed for all that is unsatisfactory. Feminists are to be thanked for the enormous amount of work they have done on mother-daughter relationships and for giving us a vocabulary and a way of thinking that can be extremely useful in helping us to think about what goes on between mothers and daughters. This chapter owes a lot to their work, especially to Susie Orbach and Louise Eichenbaum. This chapter also owes a lot to Kim Chernin. She has been particularly interested in the connection between the mother-daughter relationship and eating disorders.

MONICA'S STORY

Monica had a very difficult, troubled beginning to her life. She had had to grow up much too quickly and had played a role in her family far beyond her emotional capacity. For her the complication lay in the fact that her father had divorced her mother and that her mother was left penniless looking after a handicapped son who would never be able to live alone. Now Monica had plenty of rage and plenty of unmet need to deal with in relation to her mother, but she also saw that her mother was herself extremely hungry and empty and that her life was very unhappy. How could Monica go off and be happy, contented, successful, when her mother was so unhappy and deprived? I think it is not exaggerating to say (as Monica eventually said herself) that she was determined not to be happy. The way she chose to be unhappy (or one of the ways) was to have an eating disorder. It prevented her from being successful in her work because it led to absences; it got in the way of her relationship with her boyfriend because it could be so preoccupying; it prevented her from enjoying the way she looked (and she was beautiful) because it made her look and feel terrible; it stopped any possibility that she might think well of herself because she so hated and despised herself for misusing food.

Now what is the sense in an unhappy mother's misery being equalled by the unhappiness of her daughter? How will that help or make things better? In ordinary everyday logic, of course, it will not, but at one level it made good sense to Monica. To her being happy and successful felt like an attack on her mother, felt like abandoning her, even killing her. Her answer to this dilemma was that she would be unsuccessful and she used her eating disorder to make her so. She was identifying with her mother.

How could this shift or change? What could get Monica out of this dilemma? Part of what was going on, and it is not uncommon in women who have had to grow up too quickly, was that Monica was confused between the adult part of her which could see her mother's need and the child part of her which had always known about it and grown up quickly in order to try to look after it. On a rational adult basis it was true that Monica's mother was not in a very good situation. She was miserable, short of money and trapped by the needs of her handicapped child. On the other hand, the best way for Monica to help her, again on a rational basis, might well have been for her to be as successful as possible so that she would have some money that she could give to her mother. And as to her mother's misery, Monica knew rationally that her mother had always been miserable, that she, Monica, had never been able to help her mother to be happy in the past and that she was unlikely to be able to do so now. Monica would do very well if she sorted out her own problems and miseries. She could not save her mother's soul for her, although it was sad that it was so.

It seemed that Monica was much more in touch with the part of her which perceived her mother's situation with the eye of the s nall child catapulted too soon into adult responsibilities. She felt that she was being asked to take care of her mother's needs (and historically she probably was). What the child part of her could not see then and could not see now was that those demands were inappropriate and impossible. Neither as a child nor as an adult was it possible for her to make her mother happy. None of us can take responsibility for another person's happiness. Our happiness is our own responsibility.

CAROLINE'S STORY

Caroline's mother had come to Britain from abroad as a young woman and had never reconciled herself to the loss of her own mother and exile from her native land. She was a miserably depressed woman and again Caroline grew up far too quickly in her attempt to take care of her mother. Caroline's anger with her mother was, however, much more obvious than Monica's and at 16 she left home for good, deaf to her father's advice that she should do A Levels. She desperately wanted to be out of an environment in which her mother seemed to demand everything and give nothing. She was furious with her mother for being such a victim.

However, although Caroline's anger had blasted her out of her family home, it could not blast her mother out of her head. Caroline worried a lot about her, desperately wanted to make her happy, felt terribly guilty about abandoning her. And again, like Monica, she felt she must not be happy and successful herself. Her preoccupation with food made sure that she never felt confident about herself, prevented her from having boyfriends, reduced her capacity to work effectively and gave her reason to hate and despise herself.

For both of these women there was a lot of hate and anger in the way they treated themselves. This is often the case for food misusers and then the hate and anger that they are directing against themselves is what they feel for other people. Both Monica and Caroline were in a rage with their mothers as well as identifying with them in their pain, but neither of them could acknowledge that fact. After all, how could these two women be angry with mothers so pathetic and so miserable? Instead they violently attacked themselves.

In a way, however, they were also attempting to fill the hole inside themselves left by mothering that had not been good enough. They were trying to respond to needs within themselves that had never been recognised or met.

In reality neither of them had been able during their growing up to express the hate and anger that we all have in a good situation, let alone in a bad one. Their mothers gave them no help in dealing with these feelings and so they both learned not to know about them and to translate them into the language of food. Both of them had a lot of work to do thinking about their mothers. For

Monica that had to be done with me. Her mother was simply not capable of talking about what had gone on between her and Monica. Caroline was able to work quite a lot with her mother. There was a lot of shouting and crying, but it ended up with Caroline having a much better relationship with her mother and much less of a problem with food.

COMPETITION BETWEEN MOTHERS AND DAUGHTERS

There are other ways, however, in which women find the relationship with their mothers so difficult that they resort to eating disorders. One is the whole area of competition and success. It is usual to think about men's difficulties with success in terms of the relationship with their fathers: 'Am I as good as Dad? Can I be as successful and not feel I am attacking him? Can I be successful without guilt? Do I have to make sure that I am less successful for fear of his envy?' and so on. But these issues are very much around for women and their mothers too, although it is often more difficult to detect because competition between women is so little acknowledged. On the whole women seem to find such difficulty with the idea of competition that they even deny it exists. They can do this in numerous ways, of which the most obvious is simply to refuse to compete. The refusal to compete stems from a fear equally of success or failure, but it is not that they are not competitive; it is that they are afraid of competition. Now this is not to say that women do not have great talent for collaboration. The women's movement particularly has shown that women can co-operate successfully to achieve a common goal. However, women perhaps don't help themselves by failing to know much about their competitiveness.

One of the moments when this question of competition can arise is at puberty. As daughters we are no longer children but developing young women. It is a commonplace that this often happens just as our mothers are nearing the end of their procreative lives. It can be very painful for a woman who is conscious of the ageing process really taking hold – on her skin, her muscle tone, her energy levels – to be faced with a nubile young body and a flirtatious young woman where it seems that only yesterday there was a grubby little girl. Daughters are often acutely aware of their mother's feelings and may decide that it is just not safe or possible to offer a challenge. The obvious way to sidestep the issue is for the daughter to cease to offer competition by getting either fat or very thin and thus defer the whole issue of competition.

This way of competing with our bodies and our appearance is also felt to be very dangerous because, as feminists have helped us to recognise, women's sense of themselves, their feelings, their identity are all almost inseparable from their bodily awareness. For many women their capacity to like themselves depends very heavily on how they look. This does not seem to be the same for men. They seem much more readily to be able to value themselves as distinct from the way they look. So there occurs that phenomenon that so enrages women that a fat man who stinks of B.O. will make a pass at a woman. How dare he feel that he is all right and acceptable when he is so ugly and smells bad?

The competition between fathers and sons often seems to be carried out in action, in who can win. So boys compete with their fathers to win at tennis, at chess, at making money and in finding sexual partners (just like mother). These limited areas of competition probably have the advantage of not seeming to lay everything on the line: 'Well, he may be able to beat me at tennis, but I know a lot more than him about the Stock Market.' The danger of the competition between mothers and daughters, perhaps, is that it seems to be about who we are, about everything. If as daughters we sense our mothers can't stand the competition, or if we ourselves feel unready to take it on, we may have to take evasive action. One way of doing that is to gain or lose weight.

Weight gain at this age and stage is so common that we even have a name for it – 'puppy fat'. Of course there is an ordinary and appropriate weight gain at this stage of our development brought about by hormonal changes, but our difficulties in becoming very obviously our mother's rival may well have something to do with considerable weight gain or loss.

However there can also be difficulties of competition between daughters and mothers over accomplishment and achievement, just as there are between sons and fathers. One client of mine had a mother who was an extremely successful musician. Her daughter, Hilary, was herself talented in several artistic fields, as a singer, a dancer, an actress (but not, interestingly, as a musician). From childhood it had been expected that she would do something very remarkable as a performing artist. Her chief interest when I knew her was in dance, but she was prevented from becoming anything like as good as she might have been by her eating disorder which was so severe and had gone on for so long that it seriously threatened her health. By vomiting and laxative abuse she had so much depleted her body of vital minerals that her health was severely undermined. This stopped her dancing. The issue seemed to be whether, with such a distinguished mother and such expectations of her, Hilary could dare to compete.

Much more often our mothers have accomplished very little in any professional or career sense. This can nonetheless place a heavy burden on us, for anything we accomplish in that way will surpass their achievement. Perhaps we fear their envy, fear our own wish to do better, and that may be partly why so many women finish a training or an education and then do nothing with it. Many women seem to use eating disorders to get themselves out of training or education. It seems an awful lot safer to fail, and interestingly mothers are the ones who say, 'Never mind. I just want you to be happy.' Fathers tend to say, 'I think you should finish the year.'

THE LEGACY OF ANGER

There is also the question of the rage about their mothers that so many women carry with them. Some of that is probably built in. Mothers are extremely powerful in the lives of young children and it would be an extraordinary child who did not have a legacy of anger and dissatisfaction. Indeed it is probably necessary for mothers to fail their children to some degree, to be unsatisfactory, or otherwise girls would never leave home. But many women seem to have the memory of real and significant bad treatment and don't know what to do with the feelings they retain from those times. They have great difficulty with their rage with their mothers and often direct it against themselves. You may remember the story of Isobel who got back at her mean mother by gorging packets of biscuits.

Another woman, Susan, had been trained up from an early age to be a dancer. When she was a child and teenager her mother, who was significantly overweight, had deprived Susan of food to keep her thin for dancing: 'No, Susan, no ice cream for you. Have an apple.' Mother had wanted to be a dancer herself and it looked as though Susan had the job of being both thin and a dancer for her mother. Not surprisingly this created enormous rage and resentment in Susan, but while she was at home she was too frightened to be able to express it, although there were lots of rows about food and Susan's secret sweet eating. When she left home she began to put on weight to such an extent that her ability to go on dancing was at risk. There was tremendous secret satisfaction for Susan in seeing how she could enrage and pay back her mother for what she had put her through simply by eating the things she had been deprived of for all those long years. It was some time before she could see that, however, and even longer before she could separate out whether it was only her mother who wanted her to dance. Her fury with her mother was bringing her to destroy her dancing before she had really considered whether she might like it for herself.

One woman whose beginnings had not been happy had a mother who was so bossy and interfering that she would even demand that her daughter talk when mother thought she should. Of course that created a real game between them when Theresa discovered she could wind her mother up just by not saying anything. There was a lot of real unhappiness for Theresa which she dealt with by getting very thin. In due course she left home and when she went back to visit used to raid the refrigerator and eat voraciously. It seemed as though she was trying to express all her hatred and anger with the mother who didn't love her well enough, by stealing and spoiling other kinds of nourishment.

THE NEED TO SEPARATE

Some perspective on all these examples of mother/daughter relationships can be gained if they are placed in the context of what is the major issue for mothers and growing daughters: that of separation. The question for all mothers is, 'Can I let my daughter go with my blessing to live her life as well as she can and for herself?' The question for all daughters is, 'Can I let my mother go and live as well as I can and for myself?'

Often when people hear the word 'separation' they seem to imagine some final parting, some absolute ending. Indeed, men have often been praised for what is seen as their ability to leave their mothers behind them and go off and live their lives. More recently, however, people have begun to wonder whether men's much vaunted independence comes from an organic process of emotional growth, or from a cutting off and denial of feelings. It is becoming ever clearer that men rely on women to do all kinds of emotional work for them, and by that means avoid much of the pain of feelings. On the other hand, women have often been criticised for failing to separate and for holding on to what seems an inappropriately 'childish' role in relation especially to their mothers. For instance I heard a conversation on the bus one day where a couple in their sixties were describing their grown-up daughter, married and with children. What they described was a total dependency: 'She phones up and she's round to us for the least little thing. If anything happens,' said her mother, 'she wants me to be round to her.' It seems as though in this case no psychological separation whatever has taken place. On the other hand, recent thinking has suggested that independence and individuation for women is not and probably will never be the kind of ruthless detachment that men so often seem to practise. Women have in their growing up developed an ability for connectedness which is a strength and of great importance.

So then, what does it mean to talk about women separating from their mothers? It means mothers and daughters reaching an understanding that they are two separate individuals. At one level, of course, this is blindingly obvious, but at another it is not. They are not separate if the inner and emotional lives of mother and daughter are still tangled up together. In all the situations that were described earlier this was the case. All of those daughters were behaving in ways that were to do with their mothers rather than with themselves. They were unable to be clear about what they wanted and what was for their good as distinct from their mothers'. In a way they were living in this respect as if they and their mothers were the same person, a single unit, unseparated.

The issue of separation for women is a complex one – too complex to explore in detail here except for two points. One is that it demands from us a process of mourning and letting go. The mourning is for what has been good and belongs to a stage of our life now over and also for what has not been right and for what we have not been given. A lot of our holding on is in the hope that we will finally get what we feel we never had enough of: love, approval, whatever it might be. A lot of women I have worked with have returned over and over again to bad situations and come away battered. The revisiting is in the unconscious hope that this time it will be different: 'This time I will get what I want; this time my mother will be the way I want her to be.' But we also need to mourn the ending of a part of our lives and a stage of our development in order to be able to take on the challenges of adult life. The letting go has to be a mutual process. Separation is a two-way street, with some sadness in it for both mother and daughter.

The other point is that eating disorders inhibit the vital process of separation because they blot out feelings. This means that such women get stuck in acting out their feelings about their mothers and this prevents them from developing as human beings.

8

Eating your heart out

'I eat only to fill the hole in my heart.'

Compulsive eater

So far several possible meanings have been explored that singly or in combination may be at the root of an eating disorder. They have been considered as a response to crisis, as a reaction to the social role demanded of women, as a holding pattern in dealing with sexuality and growing up, as a means of self-assertion in a life that feels over-controlled by others and as a means of coping with the relationship with our mothers. However there are other ways of understanding these problems. One of these is based on the premise that both the ravenous craving that results in compulsive eating and the violent denial of hunger that results in anorexia can be physical expressions of terrible emotional emptiness that there seems no way of soothing or satisfying.

The roots of this hunger, this emptiness, are most often to be found in early experience that has not been good enough to enable a person to grow up with a full feeling of being loved and valued. Jennifer was a young woman whose childhood had been spent between her mother and her grandmother. At the age of 3 family circumstances had meant that her mother could no longer look after her and she had been sent to live with her grandmother. This in itself was bad enough since other children in the family stayed with her mother, but her grandmother was also a harsh and unloving woman with whom Jennifer was very unhappy. Now Jennifer was also a person of considerable strength and determination. She survived this beginning and used her anger about it to make a success. On the outside she appeared a cheerful, well organised and ambitious young woman. On the inside, however, there was a part of her that was a desperately unhappy and unloved child. When that part of her was touched by some incident during the day she would be overcome by the most appalling cravings and feelings of emptiness. Jennifer felt these to be a craving for food and would binge voraciously and desperately, but at the same time she would know with part of her that it was not food she was hungry for but something else.

That something else is often identified as sex. Penelope was a young woman whose parents had separated when she was quite small. The children had stayed with their mother who had remarried. By this second husband she had had other children. Penelope was violently jealous of these half-siblings because she felt rejected by her mother. As a teenager she went off in a rage to live with her father, but he too had remarried and Penelope could not make a relationship with his second wife and other children. The poor girl felt she had no parents and no home. At that time when she was quite young, only about 16, she found a boyfriend. He was a capable, successful and gentle man a few years older who was prepared to take care of Penelope. What neither one of them was prepared for was the weight of dependency that Penelope very soon began to place on him. Adam became the absolute centre of her universe. She resented his absence at work, but even more his absences when he went to play squash and meet his friends. She had an insatiable need to be cuddled and comforted and attended to by him. This need was often felt to be sexual so that a great deal of love-making went on between them. Nevertheless sex left her feeling empty and unsatisfied, wanting more – although she could not identify what that 'more' was.

Adam told Penelope that he felt that if she could, she would get right inside him. During his absence this emptiness, this craving, could become unbearable and would be experienced by Penelope as a compulsive need to eat. She would then binge and vomit. At other times she would protect herself from these feelings by total self-sufficiency and in these moods would triumphantly do all sorts of things that she was usually afraid to do on her own. At these times she would also stop eating.

What Penelope was in touch with was the painful truth that her relationship with her boyfriend could not satisfy needs that dated from much earlier in her life. With part of her she was a baby needing a mother; a sexual relationship touched on those same needs for intimacy, dependency, loving and holding, but because she was not in fact a baby with her mother, but a young woman in a relationship with another young adult, those needs could never be properly satisfied. An adult sexual relationship is not, so to speak, designed to do that job, although it can certainly from time to time satisfy some of the residual infant needs of an adult. For the same reason, and much more obviously, infant needs cannot be met by bingeing. On the other hand, those infant needs cannot be denied by starvation – or at least not without paying a price so high that it makes nonsense of starvation as a way of coping.

THE LIFE-LONG INFLUENCE OF CHILDHOOD EXPERIENCES

This approach rests heavily on the assumption that the way things were for us when we were very small and during our growing up has a very profound effect on us in our adult lives. This is not the book or the place for a demonstration of this theory, although much of what is said here owes a lot to the object relations theories of human development, in particular as expressed by D. W. Winnicott and those who have since developed his ideas.

(References to their work will be found in Chapter 10.) All the evidence suggests that early experience has a very profound effect on us, for good or ill, and that much though we might like to we cannot forget about it, because it affects us powerfully all the time in the way we live our adult lives. It is as though that early unhappiness lives and is active inside us. We can find that we respond to situations as if we were still terrified babies or needy or neglected children of six or eight or ten. We might want to forget, but in all kinds of ways our earlier distress will make itself known.

For some people early deprivation will find expression in their lives as adolescents and young adults in the form of eating disorders. People who have eating disorders and come to me for counselling often ask, 'Why now?' 'If it is true,' they say, 'that the root of my problem was in all the awful things that happened while I was growing up, why has it taken until now, when I am 18 (or 20 or 22) for it to become a problem? Why didn't I have an eating disorder then, when it was all happening?' This is a difficult question to answer. It appears that some children actually do not manage to cope with the difficulties of their childhood and become disturbed to such an extent that they become obviously emotionally ill – occasionally with eating disorders. However, most children seem to find ways of coping with whatever is not good enough in their family environment until their mid- to late teens. At that point several things happen. One is that most leave home; another is that they begin to enter into important relationships with potential partners; a third is that they make the radical change from school to college or work. This period – which might take place any time within the decade or so between 16 and 25 – is a time of great stress and change. If there is not a firm foundation on which to build, this is the moment when it will become apparent.

It is important for those of us for whom life falls apart in our late teens or early twenties to be able to recognise that we did the best job we could in surviving what was not good in our child-hoods. If we need to do some repair work it is hardly surprising and not something that should be a source of shame. We did not create the difficulties of our early lives; it was not Jennifer's fault that her mother could not look after her, or that her grandmother was cruel and unloving; it was not Penelope's fault that her parents divorced and remarried and that Penelope was faced with tremendous difficulties in knowing where she belonged. The task that lies before us when our ways of coping stop working is to try and repair some of that early damage.

A SIGNAL FOR CHANGE

The sign that time for repair work has come for some people is an eating disorder. Why? Why should that symptom have anything to do with what has gone on for us as children and growing up? The answer may lie in the associations of food and eating that were discussed in Chapter 2. The links between feeling physically full/empty and emotionally full/empty are extremely close, so close that many of us cannot tell the difference between them. We cannot tell the difference between emotional anguish and hunger; we cannot tell the difference between denying our physical hunger and denying our emotional emptiness. We eat to fill the hole in our hearts. We translate into eating behaviour all the painfulness of our emotional state. So we can try and satisfy our emotional emptiness by eating food we don't want, then angrily deny our need for love by forcing food out of our bodies, then furiously refuse to acknowledge that we need love or people at all by starving ourselves and cutting ourselves off from the feelings of hunger and of need.

But why is it all so complicated? If we translate emotional hunger into physical hunger or our fear of love into denial of hunger, why don't we just do that? Why don't we just get on with it, if that's our answer? In fact some (fortunately few) people do just get on with it. They literally eat or starve themselves to death. For them the translation of what is emotional into what is physical works all too well. But for the vast majority of us, our solution to the problem turns out to be no solution at all. For a start it isn't complete. Try as we might to deal with our pain by our eating behaviour, we still remain aware of our pain. Penelope tried to blot out her craving for Adam's presence by eating, but she found herself still with the pain of her longing and the living hell of her eating disorder as well.

Often the problem for those with backgrounds of early deprivation is *not* simply that they want to be loved and cherished. The problem is that they want to be loved and cherished, but that simultaneously they are terrified that those who say they love them in fact do not, and will betray them. The meaning they make of their early experience is that their trust and love was betrayed. They think it is much too dangerous to love. They want to, some of the time, but they get terribly frightened, so frightened that they retreat, back off, withdraw, or attack and destroy. In fact they are so frightened that they do not consciously know much about this process in emotional terms at all. Instead they experience it, they live it, in terms of food and eating. They live their emotional lives in terms of food.

The pain of this way of living is horrific. It is a living torment that has no end. The despair and lack of hope that there is in such a way of life is a nightmare. Women say to me hopelessly 'I can't see how it will end. I can't see any way out.'

But I think that in that very hopelessness and despair there is hope. When people begin to recognise that their eating behaviour takes them nowhere except to more pain and more agony, then they may begin to be willing to consider whether there is another solution, another way to live their lives. While they believe that eating behaviour is the way to solve their problems there is little that anyone can do for them. But once they can begin to hear the whisper of doubt in their minds, then there is a chance that they will start to look for a better way to live their lives. Nothing changes overnight however. No one that I know has had a conversion from an eating disorder that has instantly solved the problem, but a lot of people I know have gradually and, often a bit reluctantly and unwillingly, started off on the road to a more satisfying way to live.

So what am I suggesting? I am suggesting that eating disorders are not only hell in themselves but that there is no hope in them. They do nothing for us; in fact they do worse than nothing — they actually compound our misery. We may therefore come to that point where we are willing to try an alternative that might have some hope attached to it. In my view that alternative is to begin to think and feel about our beginnings, our early experience, our past lives.

This will not be easy nor will it be painless. In fact it may well prove an exceedingly painful process. However, as has been suggested already, the pain of our underlying difficulties may not be worse than the pain of our eating disorder solution. In many situations I believe that to be true. I see lots of women for whom facing the underlying issues is a great relief. They are literally fed up to the back teeth with food misuse. The kind of feeling and crying that facing their problems arouses in them may be painful, but it is nothing in comparison to the torment of food misuse.

For those with very long-standing difficulties of early deprivation there is no guarantee that the pain of knowing about all that will be less. It may be just as bad as they fear. However it does have two very valuable hopes attached to it. One hope is that facing the past will bring an end to the eating disorder, and the other is that it is a process that will accomplish something much more fundamental: it will enable them to lay the ghosts of the past to rest. Eating disorders have no hope and no end.

If you recognise yourself in all this, it is very likely that you are going to need some help. Chapter 11 includes a description of the kind of help there is available, but let me tell you first how it went for one young woman with this kind of very difficult problem to resolve.

ANGELA'S STORY

The first public sign of Angela's falling apart was her failure to come to college. It was not the hiccup in attendance that is experienced by anyone who has an ordinary bad day, but the paralysing inability for weeks on end to get into college for more than one or two days a week. She was fortunate in a way that she was a student at a dance school. In such institutions there is a great stress on attendance because improvement depends on consistent, regular, daily work. Her absence was noted as it might not have been had she been following some other course of study. She was urged to find some help and because there was a bit of her that was frightened and wanted to get better she did.

As she started to talk it became clear that Angela's public statement of her difficulties by her absence had come at the end of a long period of great pain and misery. At this point it was not at all clear what lay behind her distress, but what was obvious was the torment in which she had lived for at least a year. Angela was bulimic. When the craving to eat came upon her she would stuff herself with whatever she could find until her abdomen was distended and painful. Then she would make herself sick. Exhausted by all this she would fall asleep. In a really bad episode she could spend days and nights like this, losing all sense of time. She would become possessed by a violent sense of anger and self-hatred – since she was so vile and horrible she deserved bad treatment and punishment. Once she began to binge and feel disgusted with herself, she was overtaken by a frenzy of hatred for herself that locked her ever tighter into her eating and vomiting.

When it was all over, she would feel physically exhausted and emotionally devastated. She would sleep and wake up feeling it had been the most horrific bad dream. But the battered state of her digestive system, the bags under her eyes, the foul taste in her mouth were evidence that this was no dream. She was ashamed to be with people when she looked so bad. Her abdomen was swollen; fluid retention made her whole body puffy. There was no way she could put on a leotard and do her dance classes. So she stayed away from school. Sometimes she would then move into an anorexic phase and within a day or so would begin to feel strong and in control so that she could return to school. Sometimes she would spend the day in bed reading compulsively so that she need not think about anything; sometimes, as she read, she would eat biscuits, not acknowledging to herself what she was doing until she again felt sick and bloated.

Not surprisingly there was very little room for ordinary life in this way of living. There was certainly no room for a sexual relationship; there was barely room for friendships. Angela had this terrible guilty secret about food and what she did with it. She felt very, very ashamed and she judged and condemned herself, and she imagined that anyone who knew would do the same. She could only be with her friends when her eating felt under control, which was less and less often. In any case social occasions very often involved eating and drinking, so they were themselves difficult. When Angela wasn't actually bingeing, her hope and intention was to eat nothing, so going out for a meal with her friends held nothing but terror for her. Not surprisingly her friends felt upset and rejected by her behaviour and gradually had less and less to do with her. Bit by bit she became more and more isolated and more and more preoccupied with food. It was at this point that she began the pattern of absenteeism that finally brought her to somebody's attention.

Whatever was all this torment about? Well, for some considerable time Angela felt that it was about itself. In other words the problem for Angela lay in the eating disorder and the consequences that followed from it. However incomplete this view may be, it does need to be treated with respect for two reasons. One is that there is the possibility of physical illness causing these symptoms and that possibility, however small, needs to be eliminated. Angela's visit to the doctor revealed a body suffering from the brutal punishment that it had been given, but otherwise healthy. Secondly, any person with an eating disorder has before her the preliminary task of consciously acknowledging that there is a problem. It is not for nothing that Alcoholics Anonymous insists on members publicly acknowledging the difficulty whenever they speak in a meeting: 'My name is X; I am an alcoholic.' Until a person with an eating disorder is able to recognise consciously what she is doing to herself, she is unlikely to be able to stop.

When a person with an eating disorder seeks help in counselling or therapy, she needs the opportunity to discover that she will not be treated with the contempt and judgement that she doles out to herself on a daily basis. Unless there can be that much safety and acceptance, she is most unlikely to say any more about anything. Gradually Angela began to be able to trust the counselling space and to allow us both to know about a lot of awful things that had happened to her and that still bothered her a great deal.

This was a painful process. Sometimes Angela lost sight of me as someone who was on her side. I became the judging, condemning, rejecting person that she was so often to herself. For a long time whenever she had a binge she would stay away because she imagined that I was going to hate, attack and despise her for it, the way she hated, attacked and despised herself. She was in a nasty tight corner. With part of her she needed and loved and trusted me, but with another part she was terrified of that dependence and really frightened that I was not her friend as she sometimes thought and believed, but her judge and her tormentor. It took a long time for that to change.

What family background had produced this much fear and

how could Angela's eating disorder be understood? What was it for? How was it supposed to help? The answers to these questions emerged slowly and gradually. Angela was the eldest of four children. Her parents had married when they were still only teenagers and Angela had been born within the year. Two other girls had soon followed and then after a gap of three years there was a boy. Her mother herself had had a less than wonderful start in life which made the considerable difficulties of dealing with a baby while she herself was still not 20 even worse. The arrival very soon afterwards of other children made for what would be a challenge to the most secure and stable woman.

It was not possible to know very much about what happened in Angela's babyhood and up to the age of about 5, but from what Angela did remember and had been told, by the time she went to school she was a precociously independent little girl. She behaved like someone of 5 going on 15. From the beginning she took herself to school, went to the local shops, looked after her younger siblings. How was this premature abandonment of babyhood and childhood to be understood? It seemed probable that with some part of her Angela did not believe that she was allowed to be a baby or a little girl with needs appropriate to her age. And presumably she had come to this conclusion because in fact her over-stretched mother found it difficult to respond to those needs. Angela's mother needed this eldest child of hers to grow up almost as soon as she was born and Angela had done what she could to oblige.

But there was a further complication. The second child, also a girl, Mary, was from the beginning 'difficult' which meant that she protested and complained a great deal. Whatever attention was available from Angela's mother was hogged by Mary. Even as the babies grew a bit older Angela did not benefit. If anyone's baby needs were going to be attended to, Mary made sure it would be hers.

There was not even much to be hoped for from Angela's father.

The frustrations and difficulties of his life combined to make him explosively bad-tempered. His violent rages were often directed at Angela who was terrified by him. At the same time, in other moods he would talk to Angela, then about 12, about the difficulties in his relationship with her mother. Eventually she was also the one who was told about his affair. She was, of course, sworn to secrecy. This combination of seductive excitement in the relationship with her father, alternating with fear of his rages, was not at all easy to deal with.

How was Angela going to cope with all this? She was an intelligent child with a powerful personality so she survived what might have destroyed anyone not so strong. She became the strong, capable, cheerful one in the family. That, of course, made life easy for her family, but it left Angela extremely isolated. There was no one, and never really had been anyone, who could respond fully to her emotional needs. She learned very early to take care of herself and her own needs. As she got into her teens her friendships with both boys and girls were usually based on Angela's capacity to look after them. In the only important relationship with a boy things worked out well while Angela remained cheerful and capable. When the desperately deprived child part of her peeped out, her boyfriend responded with fear and outrage. Angela's fear that no one would ever be able to tolerate her baby needs seemed once more to be proved true.

It was probably the breaking up of this relationship combined with the move away from home to college which sparked off Angela's eating disorder. Another young woman might have had a breakdown or become very depressed. Angela began a pattern of food misuse which fitted in with the needs of her family for her not to be overtly demanding. Food was the 'feeder without feeling', the inanimate mother to meet her needs. By this time she had in any case learned her lesson well and had discovered how not to let *herself* know about her emotional needs. So at that point it did not seem to her as though a lot of problems from the past had

finally caught up with her. It seemed rather that she was myste-
riously unable to control her weight. She was starting on the path
that finally brought her to seek some help three years later.

How could all of this be helped? Well, for one thing there was
a lot of crying to be done and a lot of anger to be expressed.
Throughout her life Angela had either repressed these feelings or
more recently expressed them in food misuse. As she grew more
able to believe that I could stand her feelings, she began to believe
she could bear them too. Feelings could be expressed and shared
with less fear of damaging or disastrous consequences to either of
us. Inevitably that meant she had less need to misuse food; she did
not need her inanimate feeder any more and the strength began to
ebb away from that compulsion.

Secondly there was a lot of thinking and feeling and understanding for us to do together about how Angela's early life had
influenced her. It was not only that on any objective scale her
growing up had taken place in difficult circumstances – that certainly needed to be remembered and pondered. What was also
important was to understand what Angela had made of all that.
For example, Angela believed (without consciously knowing it)
that her mother had not been able to bear her feelings (which
was probably true) and that *therefore* no one else could either.
Consequently she had to take care of them herself. Was that true?
Was it true as far as I was concerned? And if it was not true for
me, might it be that it was not true for other people either? This
enquiry had direct bearing on Angela's eating disorder because it
opened the way towards the possibility of trusting and mutual
relationships in which the feelings and needs of both parties could
be acknowledged. The need for the lonely and isolated eating
behaviour solution became less acute.

But there was a further and very important process at work as
Angela and I continued to talk. I became very important for
Angela because I was able to do and be for her a person of a kind
she had never experienced enough of before. I listened to her, I

focused on her, I thought about her and remembered her when we were not together, I attended to her and in so doing recognised and validated her as a precious human being. I did not do any of this perfectly, or without mistakes or lapses, but I did it better than it had been done for her before. In an important way I became a mother for Angela, since that is what ordinary good mothers do – they attend to their children's emotional (and physical) needs.

As our relationship continued and deepened Angela became more able to believe that I would be available to her emotionally when she came to see me. This had important practical effects in making her eating disorder less necessary, but it also created something different in the way Angela could be to herself. One way of saying it would be like this: Angela's mother had in some important ways not been good enough for Angela so Angela had never had modelled to her ways of being good to herself. She was as careless and neglectful of her own feelings as her mother had been – indeed probably considerably more careless and neglectful. But I was not careless and neglectful of her feelings. On the contrary, to the best of my ability I gave them close and careful attention. Gradually Angela learned to do the same. She too came to believe that what went on inside her was worthy of attention and respect. She began to be able to pay attention to the screams and yells of the infant/child part of herself.

What that meant was that although there was quite a long period of time in which Angela dared to feel quite dependent on me – and therefore vulnerable to the pain of absence between sessions and during holidays – yet she was engaged in a process of growth which gradually enabled her to develop her own good mother inside her and so have less need of me. By that time the kind of attack on herself that bingeing, vomiting, starving had been was no longer part of the way she treated herself.

At that point Angela came to the end of her course and therefore to the end of our time together, since I was the student counsellor. We had worked for almost three years, mostly once a week, during the most difficult time twice a week, and in occasional times of crisis more often. We had accomplished a great deal together. Neither of us would say it had been easy, painless or at times even pleasant. There had been no inevitable trajectory of progress. Rather there had been quite a few bumps, lurches and hiccups. Furthermore, neither of us believed that Angela was now beginning on a pain-free existence. On the contrary, she was beginning a life in which she would be free to feel her pain instead of translating it into eating behaviour. Nor had we together dealt with all the issues that were difficult for Angela. If circumstances had permitted we might have gone on longer. But in a way we had done enough. Angela was ready to leave home in a way that she had not been ready to leave her parental home. She wanted to try her wings and she had some confidence that this time they would be strong enough to let her soar.

This is all now several years ago. I see Angela from time to time. In some areas of her life things have gone pretty well. She is developing her professional career with some success. She has had some painful relationships which I am delighted to hear have made her very unhappy, delighted that she has become capable of ordinary human unhappiness rather than the grinding misery of an eating disorder. I am sure that the process of emotional growth will continue in her and I have some confidence that she will find herself a partner with whom she can have a mutual and caring relationship.

So where does that leave you, the reader? I hope it does not leave you thinking that a miracle was accomplished for Angela. It was no miracle; it was the result of a lot of hard work over a long period for both of us. It gives you an idea of just how much effort goes into trying to deal with and mend things that have not been good enough in our early lives. Sadly, there is no magic.

Secondly, things don't always go easily. Angela and I had a fairly bumpy ride together. Sometimes it doesn't work out and the therapeutic relationship comes to a premature end. Maybe for that person only so much could be accomplished at that time with that counsellor and more will be possible later. Rosie was someone who found the whole process of looking at what her bingeing and laxative abuse might be about unbearably painful. She wanted to think about it, but it was at that time just too awful. She tried over quite a long period of time, but it was too hard. She left the school and I lost track of her. Two years later I met her quite by chance and she told me that she had found a therapist with whom she had been working for the past six months and that things were beginning to come together for her. I was extremely pleased because it made me feel that although what Rosie and I had done together had not in any ordinary sense been a 'success', it had been good enough for her to feel that it was worth another try. To dare to confront the wounds of our early lives takes a lot of courage from both parties. It is a difficult and painful process, but it has some hope attached to it and food misuse has none.

9

Eating disorders as a response to sexual abuse

> Anorexia, like compulsive eating, is an attempt to protect your-
> self, to assert control . . . You are trying to regain the power
> that was taken from you as a child.
>
> Ellen Bass and Laura Davis, *The Courage to Heal*

Since this book was first written it has become very much more
obvious that many children are sexually abused, and what the
devastating emotional effects of such abuse can be. It has also
become clearer that many women use preoccupation with food,
size and shape as a way of coping with a history of sexual abuse.

In this chapter I want to discuss first of all how women that I
have worked with have used eating disorders to deal with the
memory and the fact of sexual abuse, and secondly how they
have used eating disorders to cope with the effects of sexual abuse
on their day to day functioning.

REMEMBERING BUT NOT FEELING

I have worked with a number of women who were abused as children and have never forgotten that fact, but who have used eating
disorders as a way of keeping the feelings about the abuse away
from them. These women can talk about the abuse, but it is as if
it happened to someone else.

Carla was one such person. She had been regularly and sys-
tematically raped by her grandfather over a period of years. There

had been no-one that she could tell, so she was left to deal with this awful reality on her own. She was in a terrible situation and it is not surprising that she needed some extreme way of dealing with it. For some years she transferred her anxiety and fear and disgust into the fantasy that she had syphilis. Eventually, in her early twenties, she had the courage to get herself tested and found that she did not have and never had had syphilis. But this discovery left her without a means of protecting herself from feelings that she could not yet tolerate. She 'chose' instead (but not of course in any conscious way) anorexia as another way of displacing her fears. Carla was one of those anorexics who was not so much preoccupied with counting calories as maintaining an anorexic way of life. She starved herself of food (no breakfast, no time for lunch or just a quick sandwich, dinner if her husband made it, or just a drink and a few peanuts) and she was very thin. But she also starved herself of sleep, of warmth (she didn't wear enough clothes), of pleasure (life was just work), of a social life and in fact of everything that makes life pleasurable and enjoyable. If occasionally she did allow herself some minor treat, such as lying in for an hour, she felt that she had been 'selfish', and then she had to make up for that lapse by more than ordinary efforts. This system took up every shred of Carla's energy and attention so that she couldn't possibly come in contact with the feelings relating to the abuse she had suffered. The road to acknowledging those feelings and working through them was a long one, and it began with Carla gradually being able to recognise simple feelings in her body such as tiredness and hunger. The feelings relating to the incest were so terrible that she had had to find a way of deadening herself to all feeling.

REMEMBERING AND NOT REMEMBERING

Other women whom I have worked with have had the suspicion, the feeling, the faint memory of something awful that happened.

They aren't sure what it was exactly; they worry that maybe they made it up or imagined it; it comes back to them in dreams and momentary flashbacks. But they have nothing firm or concrete to go on. Some people, therapists, judges, social workers, parents, find it easy to accuse women of 'making things up'. Children have been known to describe quite explicitly how they have been abused only to be told that they are bad for making things up. That children or women might do this has always seemed very unlikely to me. I don't find the women I work with full of fantastic invention, rather the reverse. They are concerned with finding the truth and are afraid of exaggerating or fantasising what has happened to them. I think you can take any suspicions you have that you may have been abused very seriously indeed. However, these suspicions are often extremely painful and disturbing, and women will often work hard to distract themselves from persistent worries. Eating disorders are one of the ways women use to do this.

Philippa was someone who slept very badly and had recurring dreams that woke her up in a state of panic. One of these dreams was that a man was pushing something down her throat, trying to suffocate her. She also had a whole range of 'daydreams' that came to her when she was between sleeping and waking: one was that a man was coming upstairs and into her room; another was that she was lying in bed and a man was in the same bed with her and she could feel his erect penis against her buttocks. This last was not the ordinary pleasant sexual fantasy of the grown woman, but the terrifying anxiety of the child. Were these dreams some indication of a reality that Philippa did not remember? For many years she had been too terrified of these shadows to allow herself to consider them. Instead she had filled every waking moment with worries about food, shape and size. Philippa was a compulsive eater and stuffed down her suspicions and her memories with the food she ate. Only in her dreams and half-waking state did these persistent images come back to haunt her. I was the first person to whom she had confided these suspicions and I took them very seriously. They made sense to me in terms of what I already knew about Philippa's family, and in terms of the way Philippa was in the present. We began to work on these images by saying, 'If this is an accurate memory, what do you think it means? If this is an accurate memory what was happening? If this is an accurate memory what does it explain in the present and about how you are now? If this is an accurate memory, what feelings go with it?'

By these means we began to understand more about Philippa's experience and inner world. Then she began to say, without any prompting from me, that she thought she really didn't need to binge in the way she had, so that gradually over time she gave up having to cope by bingeing.

FORGETTING

Quite often people come into counselling complaining of something, for instance an eating disorder, and feel that the complaint is the 'real' problem. This is the 'if only I were ten pounds lighter then my life would be perfect' syndrome, and it usually covers all sorts of other worries and fears. As counselling proceeds it becomes clearer what these underlying issues are, and people frequently remember all sorts of things they had 'forgotten'. So far as modern neurological discoveries can tell us it seems highly unlikely that we truly 'forget' anything. Even those experiences that date from before words and the full development of our brains seem to leave traces and feelings behind. It has for example proved well worth while for some people to attempt to imaginatively reconstruct their birth experience, of which they have no 'memory' in the most obvious sense.

When we feel safe and understood and not judged, we can have access to all sorts of memories and feelings that otherwise we keep well hidden, even from ourselves. It is in this way that memories of sexual abuse sometimes surface when they have previously not been available to conscious memory. Beverley was one such person. She had grown up in a household where there was a lot of violence and had suffered a particularly unpleasant childhood. She was a compulsive eater and had been for as long as she could remember, and apparently for a very good reason. In her twenties she joined a group for compulsive eaters and began to work on the underlying problems and difficulties in her life. She found the group helpful and through it came to the realisation that she was not alone in her compulsive eating and that she could learn from other people's memories and experience. Bit by bit she remembered many things she had forgotten from her childhood which up to that point had been very shadowy, with lots of gaps. Among other things, she gradually remembered that her father had sexually abused her from when she was still quite small, over a period of several years. There was no doubt in her mind about these memories; she remembered all kinds of details that fixed them in time and place, but up to then they had been totally absent from her conscious mind. Of course, it was not specially easy to have these things coming back to mind and Beverley got very upset about it on many occasions and for a long time afterwards. However, it was also a relief because it explained aspects of her behaviour that she had never really been able to understand before, including her fear of sexual relationships with men.

This theme of relief is not uncommon when women remember things that have been long forgotten. Hannah, like Beverley, had been physically abused as a child by both of her parents and this she had never forgotten, nor the fear and rage that went with the memories. However, she had a long history of a troubled relationship with food and size and had been first anorexic for several years, and then bulimic. When I got to know her we spent a lot of time working through her relationship with her parents. This helped the bulimia but did not really get rid of it. However when she began to remember the way her grandfather had sexually abused her she uncovered a whole area of feeling and experience that had previously been hidden. Then she began to understand more about the way she related to men in the present and more about her relationship with her parents and their relationship with their parents. This was extremely painful for Hannah, but also hailed a very creative period which brought an end to the bulimia once and for all.

SEXUAL RELATIONSHIPS AND INTIMACY WITH MEN

It is not unknown for women to abuse children sexually and it is certainly not unknown for boys to be abused, but in this chapter I am focusing on the sexual abuse of girls by men, and in this section on the effects that the abuse has in the day to day lives of those abused girls once they grow up.

Perhaps the most obvious and easy to understand of the effects of sexual abuse are the problems it causes many women in forming adult sexual relationships. These problems are often disguised for a long time by eating disorders.

One woman, a compulsive eater for many years, described herself as someone who had had 'lots of sex but not much love'. As a child she had been given sex rather than love, but of course her need as a child was for love, and not for sex. The two were hopelessly confused in her mind. Somewhere inside her she thought that if she had sex she would get love; she had been an unloved child, like most victims of incest, and had complied with the demands of her abuser in the desperate need and hope of some sort of attention. In her adult life she did the same. Out of desperate need she engaged in any sexual liaison that was on offer and again found herself unloved. Instead she found comfort the only way she knew, with food. She thought the only thing about her that anyone wanted was her sexual availability, since that was what she had been wanted for as a child, so she hid from herself with food the painful feelings of worthlessness that easily overcame her. This story has a sad ending however. This woman was in her forties; she had been living like this for twenty-five years. For her to develop would have involved an enormous change in her whole existence and way of life; it would have been a long and painful business. Evidently it seemed too difficult, at least just then, in that way, because I only ever saw her once. Maybe she went away and worked on it all on her own, maybe she found someone else to help her. I hope so.

The opposite extreme from trying to find love through sex is to abolish all thoughts of sex or interest in it. This is the solution to the trauma of sexual abuse that I have known a number of women find through anorexia. Anorexia produces a state of starvation which has the physiological effect of forcing our bodies to focus on survival, rather than reproduction. It alters a woman's hormone balance and makes her infertile – as if her body knows it cannot sustain a foetus. This combines with a lack of sexual feelings or fantasies. Not only that, anorexia is, and is meant to be, a very preoccupying state of mind. You have to work very hard to be an anorexic. You certainly haven't got the time or the energy to be thinking about sex. The only trouble with this solution is that it is a terrible way to live and an incredibly high price to pay to obliterate the trauma of the original abuse. I have known women spend all the fertile years of their lives in this state, not daring to be sexual because of that original horror and pain with which they first experienced sex.

What is commoner, at least in my experience, is for women to have sexual thoughts and feelings, but to have difficulties in actually translating those into a satisfying sexual relationship with a man. These difficulties can be disguised in various ways by eating disorders. Best known of these is: 'I feel fat and ugly. If I didn't feel like that I would be out socialising every night/settling down to a long-term relationship/looking for a sexual partner/enjoying the sexual relationship I have. However, until I have lost weight I can't do this.'

While all their attention is focused on their weight these women can avoid facing both the awful truth about the past and the awful truth about the present: that they are afraid of sexual intimacy with a man and that they have good reason to feel like that.

Sometimes these difficulties only emerge when women are actually involved in a relationship and begin to realise, often through reading, that the sexual experience they have within the relationship is not the fulfilling enjoyable experience they hear that other women have. They become aware, for example, that they don't feel anything when they are being caressed intimately, that they switch off from intercourse, that the only way they have orgasms is when they masturbate in private. Sometimes such women will then have flashbacks when they are making love, to their childhood experience. One woman I worked with had flashbacks to her brother's face which momentarily displaced her lover. Often these realisations have been held at bay for years by preoccupations with food and size.

TRUST AND CONTROL

None of these difficulties in sexual function are very easy to deal with or to resolve, especially since what lies behind them are issues of trust and control. In order to have a satisfying sexual relationship we must be able to trust our partner, and to be able to tolerate not being in complete control either of the situation or of ourselves. But by definition, the victim of sexual abuse has had her trust betrayed and has been in a situation where she was not in control but was controlled for another person's use. These issues of trust and control are often central to the emotional development of the abuse survivor.

It is part of the hard work involved in having an intimate relationship to develop trust and mutuality so that neither person in the partnership feels that they are either in control or controlled. However, the person with an eating disorder, especially the sexually abused woman, has moved the issues of trust and control away from a person and a relationship and into the arena of food. For example, a teenager with an eating disorder is not struggling directly with her problems of mistrust and control through her social contacts and friendships. She will almost certainly not be quarrelling with her boyfriend about which film they will go and see or worrying whether a friend has been gossiping behind her back. The tackling of such issues would help her develop skills of negotiation, and a sense of mutuality and trust. However, the eating disordered youngster has little or no social life, falls in with whatever someone else wants to do, instead transferring issues of trust and control on to food. What she mistrusts is the packet of cereal in the cupboard, or the chocolate bar in the shop or the ham sandwich in her stomach. She doesn't know whether these things are good for her or not, and she doesn't know whether she wants to have anything to do with them or not. She thinks about dealing with them by control but she often feels that they control her. She's not anxious about whether she should go out to the cinema with the boy next door, she's anxious about whether she should have the yoghurt that's in the fridge.

One girl who was a student nurse was a very good example of this way of doing things. Instead of having a social life she sat in her room in the hostel, always finding an excuse not to go out with her friends until they grew tired of asking. Part of her wanted to go to the disco held every Friday evening: she had plenty of fantasies about meeting boys, kissing and fondling. But she was also deeply afraid of any kind of real sexual encounter with a man because of the incestuous abuse perpetrated by her father. She couldn't, at this point, bring herself to think about these worries directly, so instead she worried about food. She made herself overweight so then she could spend all her spare time thinking about dieting and/or bingeing, rather than worry-ing about the fact she both did and didn't want to find a boyfriend who she did and didn't want to kiss her.

This same technique of displacement of worries from a person on to food happens in established relationships as well (and by no means only with those who have suffered sexual abuse). When Suzanne disagreed with her husband she didn't argue with him, she went and made herself sick. When she was worried about where he was and what he was doing when he came home late, night after night, she didn't challenge him, she binged instead.

The trouble with this system is not only that the person devel-ops an eating disorder, which is bad enough; not only that they avoid dealing with the original problem, but that they deprive themselves of the emotional experience that everyone needs to make satisfying relationships and to develop within them. It's like having a learning disorder: you truant from school because you hate reading and the truanting gets you into trouble. Nobody asks why reading has become such a problem for you, but in the meantime you still don't learn to read, which means that all sorts of other activities become impossible as well. Learning to read is not an optional extra, and neither is learning to relate. This is where counsellors and therapists can be useful, because above all the task of therapy is to create a relationship within a safe and asexual environment. The relationship with the therapist ideally becomes the practice ground for relating skills, especially trust and control, which can then be applied in the real world.

SELF-KNOWLEDGE AND SELF-ESTEEM

Of all the painful and disastrous effects of sexual abuse, perhaps the worst is the feeling of worthlessness and shame with which the victims are so often left. To abuse someone sexually is to use someone for your own pleasure and gratification without regard for the victim's feelings or needs. It is to use someone as an object, to deny them their personhood. No child can ever give 'consent' to sexual abuse, however much some abusers and some members of the judiciary might want to blame the child. No adult can deny responsibility for abusing a child by saying, 'She led me on' or 'She wanted it' or 'She never objected'. The power imbalance between a child or a teenager and an adult man is enormous and adults have a duty of responsibility towards a child not to abuse that position of power and trust.

Nevertheless, despite this, plenty of abused girls feel guilty, ashamed and responsible. They also feel made dirty and disgusting. In other words they take on the feelings and the responsibility which their abuser so often denies. The result of all this is very often a devastating sense of worthlessness. 'I feel' as many abused women have said to me, ' just like a piece of shit.'

To live your life day by day feeling that bad about yourself because you have been used by another person is a hard task. Many women try to escape the feeling by using drugs or alcohol. Others use food. The advantage of using an eating disorder in this situation is that you provide yourself with a whole way of thinking that gives meaning to your feeling of worthlessness. You feel fat and ugly and that makes sense of the devastating low self-esteem you feel.

The way out of this is not easy and not quick. It means first of all that you must get in touch with that abused child, see things from her point of view and recognise in a feeling way that what happened was not her fault and does not make her worthless or bad. Then you must begin to create and develop a clearer, firmer, stronger sense of self; that, for most women, is a long slow task. Society does not value women or children highly anyway. Women's work and women's lives are often seen as worthless. It is hard to transform your inner world when the outer world seems to echo so easily your own poor opinion of yourself. You must begin to recognise your abilities and value them; one woman I worked with began to take her ability as an organiser seriously and gradually took an increasingly important role in a voluntary organisation; another learned to value and enjoy her craft skills and took a relevant course leading to a recognised qualification; another stopped saying she was useless as a mother and began to see that in some ways she was a good mother and in other ways she could develop and improve. In this process these women gained confidence, learned more about themselves, started to feel that after all they were someone, not just a piece of shit, but a person.

Even more important is to make sure that in your relationships and friendships and also at work, you do not allow yourself to be treated badly and abusively. Too often when women have been abused they come to feel that being treated badly is normal and ordinary, and do not even feel that there is anything wrong. One of the rather powerful effects of therapy is that a woman is treated with respect. The therapist listens carefully to what she has to say, takes it seriously, wants to know about her experience and her thoughts about her life and its meaning. When a woman is not used to this kind of treatment it can provide a very strong contrast with the treatment she gets elsewhere. Sometimes this means she will leave a relationship that she begins to see is repeating the abuse of her childhood.

I would like to end this chapter with two case histories. The first is the story of a woman who had been abandoned as a child and brought up in care. Already, therefore, from a very young age she was a vulnerable child. Because of a series of misjudgments about whether she might eventually be able to return to her family, she was never offered for adoption and there was no long-term fostering arrangement made. This girl, whom I will call Amanda (which means 'needing to be loved'), therefore grew up in a series of children's homes where she was both physically and sexually abused. This gross betrayal of a vulnerable child initially made her a withdrawn and lonely girl. At sixteen she was required to leave the children's home and, with very little support, try and make her way in the world. The combined effect of all this was that she developed first anorexia and then bulimia as means of coping with an experience and an emotional history that was too much for her. When I met her she was very bulimic and not at all well as a result. It took a long time for the facts of her life to emerge. The connection between painful feelings which arose from her remembering her earlier life and the bulimia was made clear by the way that Amanda would start to talk about something she had remembered, then break off, saying that the only real problem was that she was overweight and that if only I would help her deal with that problem everything would be all right. Particularly because of the sexual abuse, Amanda was full of hatred for her body and herself, and underneath full of rage for those who had abused her. She found it hard to trust anyone, even a little, with very good reason, and the abuse made the prospect of a relationship with a man intolerably complicated and difficult. During the time I worked with her, Amanda was not able to give up the bulimia; she still needed it and was not yet ready to face the terrible disaster of her childhood without that protection. I felt she had done well to get as far as she did and she went on to get help from another source. What her story will illustrate perhaps, is the need and value of an eating disorder for a girl who has been abused, and the extent of the hard work that is necessary before she can give it up.

The other story is of a woman grossly and persistently abused by her father as a child, who developed anorexia. She married a man who was rather cold and withdrawn, whose attitude to sex was that it was a biological function, an urge in a man that had to be satisfied, but was of no more emotional significance than going to the toilet. And that is exactly how Sophie experienced his love-making, as if he went to the toilet inside her. However, having been accustomed to being abused, she did not even in a conscious way object, until she began to do some work on herself because of her anorexia. She realised then both what a hideous

trauma the abuse had been and how similar she felt her husband's love-making to be. She asked him to go with her to some couple counselling, which he did, but he was completely unable to understand what Sophie was complaining about. As he said repeatedly, he had had no complaints; the only problem was Sophie's anorexia. To absorb the fact that Sophie did have complaints seemed beyond his power. As it became clearer over a period of many months that her husband was incapable of change and that her eating disorder had some connection with their sexual relationship, Sophie gradually came to the conclusion that she no longer wanted to be in the relationship. She felt strongly enough that she deserved and wanted something better to be able to leave and to begin to build a more satisfying and less anorexic life.

The wounds of sexual abuse can heal, and the disturbance they cause in ordinary living can be overcome. Often an eating disorder has been necessary as a means of survival, but if the underlying cause can be attended to and resolved then the eating disorder will no longer be necessary and can be discarded.

SECTION THREE

How to help yourself

This section has been designed to enable you to begin to explore yourselves a little more deeply to discover what lies behind your eating behaviour and how those problems can be approached. As you have read through this book you have probably found some sections that feel more meaningful to you than others, some that ring bells in relation to your history and experience. These feelings are a good guide for where to begin thinking further about yourself.

It is frequently a painful and daunting task to begin to think about our emotional history. If it were easy you would have done it long ago and would not have needed your difficulties with food. We have many painful and difficult feelings to cope with. It can be a lot easier if you can find someone to share this emotional journey. Sometimes a member of your family will be able to help you remember parts of your history. Since these problems with food are very common among women, you may be able to find another woman who will be willing to join you in a process of exploration. More formal sources of help are described at the end of the book, but in any case try to find at least some company for this task. It is a lonely business trying to deal with the difficult parts of your life all by yourself and chances are you have already done far too much of that.

EATING DISORDERS ARE NOT ABOUT FOOD

The book you have just read is based on the idea that your eating disorder is a way of protecting you from feelings that have been more than you can stand. If you can allow yourself to deal with these feelings more directly you will find that you no longer need to use food compulsively or be obsessionally concerned with your weight, shape and size. Most sufferers do not think like this at all. Most of the time they are convinced that the 'real' problem is their weight and that if only they could lose ten pounds life would be different. However, the very fact that you have read this book means that you have at least a suspicion that it isn't quite that simple. It is that suspicion that you need to help you get out of the clutches of your eating disorder. What follows here are some exercises you can try to help develop this suspicion and increase your awareness of your inner world of feelings.

Remember that these exercises are only suggestions. I don't know you personally and therefore what follows is not necessarily exactly what you need. Feel free to work on what seems pertinent to you and in whatever way is most useful. Leave aside what feels too difficult or irrelevant.

1 Think back to the time when your eating disorder began. How old were you? What is the memory that makes you realise that at that time you were misusing food? It could be something like one of the following examples which people have given me:

Stealing money as a child to buy sweets
Buying packets of biscuits to eat on the way home from school
Going to a party and spending the whole time eating
Having someone comment on how much you were eating
Dieting and enjoying the feeling of emptiness
Reaching a diet target and deciding to continue anyway
Feeling triumphant because your family needed food but you
    didn't

Making yourself throw up after meals
Secretly buying laxatives
Planning a binge
Planning a binge and planning to throw up afterwards
Weighing yourself obsessionally
Eating without knowing when you were full
Never feeling hungry
Saying you weren't hungry when you were but didn't want to
eat

Maybe the memory you come up with won't be the very beginning of the problem, but it will very likely be some kind of indication that by then the problem was getting a grip on you.

The next part of this exercise is to connect this memory of the eating disorder beginning with what was going on in your life at the time. Here again is a list of examples that I have been given:

Got married
Father died
Left home for the first time
Sexual abuse began
Mother became mentally ill
Felt alienated from social activities of peer group
Too scared to join in teenage social life
Parents split up
Husband became ill
Child died

Some people find difficulty in isolating one event which might have triggered the eating disorder, but instead can identify a continuing situation which got too much, such as continuing conflict and distress within the family, or coping with another's illness or handicap.

2 A second way of trying to correlate your eating behaviour and
your emotional history is to chart the ups and downs of your

weight over time, against your life experience. Some people with eating disorders can't remember the fluctuations in their weight over the years, but many can. If you can, try making a chart with the history of your weight on one side of a line and the history of your life on the other. It might look something like this:

WEIGHT HISTORY	AGE	LIFE HISTORY
Normal weight.	10	Primary School.
Began to put on weight.	11	Changed school/lost friends.
School nurse said I was overweight.	12–13	Lonely/no friends/parents separating.
Put on a stone in a year. Lots of nicknames, 'fatty' etc.	14	Parents divorced.
Go to Weightwatchers – try to diet. Lose weight for a while but put it all back on.	15–16	Make friends with boy in my class. Go out with him for a while. My best friend steals him.
Start to lose weight without trying. Get close to ideal size.	17–18	Two great years at college. Do well, make friends.
Put loads of weight back on.	19	Go away to college. Mother re-marries.

If you look at this chart you can see that this young woman's weight goes up and down according to whether or not she is happy. Of course, nobody can be entirely protected from the everyday unhappinesses that are part of the human experience, but this girl has used food and weight as a barometer of her emotional world. She comes from a family that is very bad at talking about feelings, so she has had to deal with the difficulties she experiences on her own. She can't really manage that and so has found a way of using food to both protect and distract herself. What is sad is that she has spent far too many of her teenage years feeling awful about the way she looks and staying home counting calories, instead of being out and about living her life.

Very often a pattern will emerge from a chart like this of weight loss or gain in response to emotional events. Although you may have been completely unaware of it at the time, you have obviously been using food to help you deal with events in your life. True, it is very common for people to lose or gain weight in response to stress, but that is not really what we are talking about. We are talking about *not* dealing with stress but instead hiding from it by obsessions with weight and food. For a person with this kind of history of food use, changes in weight are a more obvious record of distress than the memory of the feelings. One woman told me, for instance, that she didn't remember feeling anything about a very traumatic time when she was eleven. What she did remember was eating packets of biscuits on the way home from school and how terrible it was to weigh eleven stones at the age of eleven.

3 These first two exercises have been intended to help identify the connection between your emotional history and the way you have used food in the past, but you also need to be able to make those connections in the present so that you begin to see how your eating behaviour, day to day, is influenced by your feelings and what happens in your life. So often people say to me that they have absolutely no control over their eating behaviour and, as far as they can see, it has no hidden meaning or explanation at all (other than that they have no will power). I simply don't believe that such behaviour is meaningless, but I do think it can be difficult to see the connection between feeling and acting.

Try this way of doing it. Over the course of at least a few days, preferably a week, keep a record of your eating behaviour. I don't mean keep a record of *what* you eat; I'm sure you are already obsessed with that and noting it all down won't help. What I mean is keep a record of 'eating episodes', or if you are anorexic and focused on not eating, keep a record of your 'no eating episodes'. At the same time make a note of your hunger state. You can use the scale of: very hungry, hungry, slightly hungry, not hungry, full, and note down where you are on that scale. At the same time make some kind of assessment of your feeling state, for instance, bored, depressed, confused, sad, irritable, disappointed, annoyed, jealous, lonely, etc. This is not easy to do, especially to begin with, and you may find that your initial entries look something like this:

Monday morning

No breakfast, not hungry, tired and not wanting to go to college.

11AM Ate Danish pastry with coffee; don't know whether I was hungry or not. Angry with self for eating it.

1PM Big lunch – not really hungry. Had to eat alone since friends not around. Worried about work to hand in.

However maybe after a few days the same entry might look more like this:

Monday morning

No breakfast. Woke up early worrying about work to hand in. Not sure I've done it properly.

11AM Danish pastry. Little bit hungry but still worried about work. Wish I could talk to a friend about it.

1PM Big lunch – not really hungry. Still worrying about work. Had to eat alone, felt lonely and anxious.

In the second set of entries you can see how much clearer the relationship between the eating behaviour and the feelings has become; this student is trying to deal with her anxiety about her work and has no-one around to talk to about it, so what she does is try to deal with the anxiety by not eating/eating. This, of course, will neither deal with the problem, nor make her feel good about herself.

If you are anorexic you need to discover the feelings to do with decisions *not* to eat, as well as those around eating; if you are bulimic, the feelings around vomiting or purging. If you start from the assumption that since you have an eating disorder your eating behaviour is the language in which you speak to yourself, then it will be easier to persevere by asking yourself 'What am I telling myself?' rather than letting yourself off the hook of this emotional exploration by saying things like: 'I'm greedy', 'I have no will power', 'It's just a habit I can't break', etc.

WHAT DO YOU THINK OF WHEN YOU THINK OF FOOD?

1 One of the ways of trying to recreate in an imaginative way your early experiences of feeding and your emotional experience as an infant is via guided fantasy. This is a technique which relies not so much on conscious memory as on feeling memory and unconscious knowledge to get at the emotional truth of your own history. When I do this exercise with groups of women, they often start off by saying, 'But how can I know?' or 'I can imagine anything', or 'How do I know there's any truth in what I imagine?' I believe that it is very, very difficult to imagine anything about our history that does not have some emotional truth to it, and many women who have tried this exercise have found their way to some kind of greater clarity about their own early experience. You must try it and decide for yourself

It is a little awkward to organise this exercise. Ideally you could find someone who would read slowly the text that follows so that you can sit or lie comfortably with your eyes closed and concentrate on the words and the pictures they bring to your mind. It is a very powerful exercise for many people, so I would recommend you do not do it on your own. At the very least have someone you trust with you, so that if you get upset there is someone there to support you. Don't hurry; give yourself time for pictures and feelings and memory traces to surface.

Imagine you are a baby; you are very small, somewhere between three and six months old. It is morning and you've been having a nap. You are in some kind of pram or push chair outside, perhaps in a garden or on a balcony. The sun is shining, and as you slowly begin to wake up you see the light and the moving shapes and patterns of a tree nearby. How do you feel waking up? Are you rested and content, or perhaps still tired and grumpy? As you look at the light and the tree, how are you feeling? Are you calm or anxious; comfortable or restless?. . . After a little while someone comes to get you and a face appears in front of you as you lie there. Is that your mother, or who is it? What kind of expression is on her face? Is she smiling or serious or has she some other expression? Is she maybe rushed or anxious? And how do you feel? Are you happy and eager to see her? Do you lift up your hands to her or talk to her by moving your legs? What are your reactions?. . . Then this person, let's call her your mother, bends over to lift you out of the pram. How does she do that? Does she do it gently and carefully, giving you time to realise what is going on, or does she do it efficiently and without much attention to you, or does she do it rather carelessly and roughly? And how do you react? Do you get a shock or a fright, or are you feeling safe and glad to be picked up?. . . Then, your mother carries you into the place where you live. It is time for you to be fed. How does this happen? Are you breast fed, or fed with a bottle? How does your mother feel about feeding you? Does she enjoy the closeness and contact with you and wait for you to feed at your own pace? Is she rushed and anxious about all the other things she has to do? Is she preoccupied with other things entirely so that she doesn't really focus on you? Is she anxious and scared about feeding you and worried about getting it wrong?. . . How does she hold you as she feeds you, or does she hold you at all? Does she prop the bottle up and leave you to get on with it? Do you feel warm and safe and loved and comfortable so that you can enjoy feeding, or are you tense and anxious so that you keep stopping or get pains in your tummy and cry?. . . And how much milk do you take? Who decides that? Does she let you pause and think about it and then go back to feeding, or does she put the nipple/teat back in your mouth the moment you let go of it? Are you an eager, hungry feeder or do you feed slowly? Does your mother try and make you finish the bottle or can you decide when you've had enough?. . . And then, when you have finished feeding, it is time for you to be washed and changed. Your mother takes you into the bathroom and lays you down on a mat to change your nappy and clean you up. What do you feel about this? Do you kick and protest and cry, or are you quiet and busy with your own thoughts, looking about and watching your mother? How does she change you? Is she disgusted by your nappy, by the smell and the look of it, or does she think it's all right? And what about cleaning your bottom? Does she find that disgusting? How does she do it: roughly, quickly, gently, tenderly, efficiently, clinically? What message do you get about yourself from being changed like this? Do you think she really loves you and thinks you're a wonderful baby, or do you think you really ask too much of her because she has so much else to do, or do you frighten her with all your needs? Are you a joy or a burden or an anxiety to her? Or something else?. . . When you are all cleaned up she takes you back into the living room. Now you want to play and have some conversation. Is that what happens? Does she play with you and talk to you? Are there baby books and baby toys that she shows you so that you can see colours and feel shapes and reach out? Does she play baby games of peekaboo and 'I'm going to eat this little finger' and 'I'm going to kiss this tummy'? Or are you left on your own to play while she does something else? Or are you left alone with nothing to play with and nothing to look at? How do you feel during this time? Are you calm and happy, excited, touchy, scared, bored, lonely? Or something else?. . . Then someone else comes home. Who is that and what is that person's attitude to you? Do you like that person and how do you feel about them being there?. . . Later on that day it's time for you to go to sleep. How is that done? Does your mother rock you to sleep and then put you in your cot? Does she put you in your cot quietly and gently and pat you a little until you start to go to sleep? Are you left in the dark on your own? Do you cry? Are you scared or can you relax and go off to sleep easily?. . .

When you finish hearing the guided fantasy, don't feel you have to snap out of it in a hurry. It can be very powerful to be in touch with these very early experiences. Often those who do it cry and experience strong feelings of loneliness, sadness or even rage. Give yourself time to come out of it slowly and gently.

When you are ready, maybe not even the same day, you can start to think about what it means that you had that particular set of pictures and feelings during the fantasy. What does it teach you about your babyhood and the relationship between you and your mother? Do those pictures and feelings make sense to you when you put them together with other memories and feelings about your early childhood and the relationship with your mother? In particular, what do you think you can learn from it about your relationship with food/love? Remember, for a baby, food is love. There will be a very close connection between the way you were fed and the way you were loved. Is that what you use food for now – to make up for the love you didn't have then? Or if that love was too strong and overwhelming and overpowering, do you use

not eating now as a way of freeing yourself from being controlled
by the giant figure of your mother?

Remember, you don't have to do this exercise. Use it if you
think it will help, otherwise forget it. There is also no right way to
do this or any of the exercises; they are offered only as possibilities to be used as you think best.

2 For most of us the way our families used food and their attitudes to it have been intensely important in the forming of our
   emotional responses to food. This exercise is designed to help
   you become more aware of those patterns in your experience.

Make a plan or a drawing or a diagram of the room in which your
family ate as a child. Try and visualise as much detail as possible:
the way the room looked; how things were arranged; where the
window and the door were; where the sink and the refrigerator
were, if it was the kitchen; if there was a television and where that
was. Label the places at the table where each person sat, or if you
ate around the television for example, try and remember who sat
in which places. You can write these details on your drawing.
Then, try to remember the kind of food you had, maybe dishes
you especially liked or disliked, food you had often, food that
was a treat.

You can write this information on the diagram as well. Then
try to remember what the emotional interchange was like. What
kind of mood came from different people in the family? How
was the interchange between various members of the family? You
can write words beside each person, or draw lines to indicate
who talked to whom, or use colours to show the moods and feelings. Try and think of one word or phrase to describe the
atmosphere of meal-times. Then think more carefully about yourself. Where are you in this picture? Have you shown what your
feelings were in this situation? How old were you in the picture
that you have made? Does it cover a good many years or some

shorter time? What effect did this situation have on your eating behaviour and your attitude to food at the time? Can you see how your attitude to food was affected? And what about now? Can you see how you repeat any of these feelings and attitudes? Are you still stuck in the emotional atmosphere of your family's behaviour around food and meals?

It's not just easy and pleasant to reconstruct these family situations. For many women with eating disorders family meals were occasions of great tension and discomfort. You may find yourself strongly in touch with those feelings. However, try to persevere if it is like that for you, because you are getting close to some of those emotional associations with food that cause you so much trouble in the present.

EATING DISORDERS AS A RESPONSE TO CRISIS

Here again, if you use the exercises in this chapter, remember that their only use is their usefulness to you. You don't have to do them, and you don't have to do all of them. Pick and choose what is interesting and relevant for you.

1 The first thing you need to do if you feel you are using food in a strange way that you never have done before, or are suddenly worrying about your weight and size in a way that feels unpleasantly new and obsessive, is to say to yourself, 'When did this start?' Even if you can't immediately think of any connection to anything else, sort out for yourself when it began. If your eating disorder is a response to crisis it will almost certainly have a clear beginning. And then ask yourself the next question, 'What was going on in my life then?' Probably to begin with you won't feel there's any connection. You might feel something like 'Yes, well of course, that happened (something new, different, a change) but I wasn't really much bothered by that.' But think again, and ask yourself what feel-

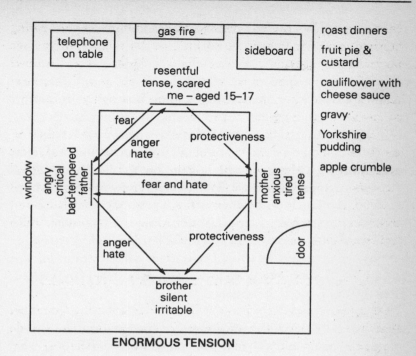

ENORMOUS TENSION

ings you had around that event and what about it hurts or upsets you still. I think you will find that there are plenty of feelings that you have been trying to deal with by your eating behaviour. So then, find someone to talk to about it – someone in your family, a friend, a teacher, a counsellor, someone you trust. These feelings have obviously been a bit too much for you and you need some time and space to sort them out.

One example I can give you of someone who responded to crisis with food was a woman whose husband became ill. There was an enormous amount of worry whether this man would ever recover, and if he did whether he would be able to work. His wife had a great deal of anxiety about the family's financial situation and tried to protect her two sons from worry. Although lots of people enquired after her husband's health, not many asked how she was managing and she didn't feel that she had the right to complain. So she turned to food, not in huge quantities, but compulsively. She put on more than a stone in weight over several months and was mortified not to be able to get into her clothes. When we started to talk about all this, she simply couldn't believe that there could be a connection between the crisis over her husband's health and her own weight gain, but gradually she could see what an appalling time it had been and how scared she had been and how lonely with her anxieties, so that she needed the little comfort that a bar of chocolate at bedtime had given her. She was a reserved, proud woman and it was hard for her to attend to her own feelings, but she could begin to see what a strain the crisis had been and even to share those feelings with her counsellor. Then she didn't need the chocolate.

If you can see that maybe some event or change must be behind your eating behaviour you may ask yourself why you had to deal with the crisis by your use of food. The answer will very probably lie in the way your family dealt with crisis and feelings and in how much support you get now from your family and relationships. One young woman identified the event that had triggered her bingeing and vomiting as a rape she had suffered some months before. Because this had happened on a date she had never reported it to the police. More surprising she had never told her family and friends. When I asked her why she hadn't told anyone, she said she thought they would say it was her fault and that she shouldn't have got into that situation in the first place. When I asked her how she knew they would say that, she said that whenever anything happened to her she got blamed for it, even if it wasn't her fault. So then this girl was used to having to deal with crises on her own, but this one had been too much for her.

Think about how your family responded to your emotional

ups and downs when you were growing up. Could you rely on them for support, or were you left to manage on your own? Maybe the way they responded was to blame or take over or to react in some way that you didn't find helpful, so you preferred to keep things to yourself. If it was like this and you have experienced something that is too much for you, it might be helpful to look for support in a new direction. Just because your family couldn't help you doesn't mean nobody else can or will.

ON BEING A WOMAN

One of the great truths about being an adult is that you can do pretty much what you want to do; you don't have to be a drudge or a victim. Whenever I say this, the women I am working with immediately contradict me and say that their lives are full of obligations, things they must do, and severe limitations on their freedom. Possibly. My sense is much more that we limit ourselves and refuse to make active choices and take opportunities; instead we hide behind what we claim that other people demand of us. Once we become adults and leave home we have enormous freedom.

1 Part of that freedom is the freedom to dream and imagine and fantasise what our lives can be. This daydreaming sometimes leads to nothing and is just a way of removing ourselves from the present reality, but it can also be the preliminary to change and development. After all, if we can't imagine change we certainly aren't going to put it into action; like the song says: 'if you never had a dream, you'll never have a dream come true.' So as a way of exploring your secret hopes and longings you might like to try some of the following exercises.

   1 An aged relative dies and leaves you £10,000. What will you do with it?

   2 You win a competition on the back of a soup tin and the

prize is six months travel. Where will you go and why?

3 You have the opportunity to train for any occupation you like. What would that be and how would you do it?

4 Imagine yourself in five years time. Where would you like to be and what would you like to be doing? Write down a description of how you would like your life to be.

5 Assume you are free of your eating disorder. What would you like to accomplish in the next twelve months?

If you find it difficult to answer these questions, then maybe you are using your eating disorder to hide from your own life and its possibilities. None of us can change our lives unless we have a vision of how we can change or to what. Eating disorders are frequently used as a way of stopping us living, and of focusing all our attention on food, size and shape, rather than how we can live creatively.

More often, though, when I have done this exercise with women, the list of dreams and hopes and fantasies has not been hard for them to make. What is sad is that it contains so much that can so easily be achieved. One woman said she would like to have long hair, another that she would like her house to be clean. If you are at all serious about your list, items like these are not hard to achieve. Other things are harder: to own your own flat, to be in a good relationship, to change your occupation. However these goals are not impossible. If you are willing to work at it you can make your dreams come true.

2 Start from the assumption that the weight and size you are at this moment is the weight and size you want to be just now. Put aside all your immediate urges to say, 'No, it isn't', and focus on the idea that there are some very good reasons to look just the way you do. What are they? Here's a list that other women have provided on previous occasions to start you off:

To defy my parents
To feel strong
To protect myself against other people, especially men
To make sexual relationships impossible
To protect a part of me that is scared and uncertain
To get me out of social situations
To show people how unhappy I am
To take revenge on those who have hurt me

Try and find other reasons of your own. When you have a list
(not necessarily a long one) that feels emotionally right, try and
think further about what you are using your size for, and whether
you can tackle those problems more directly. For instance, one of
my clients used her weight to protect her from having to
socialise; she was close to being agoraphobic. She hated the parties and gatherings that went on at work and did her best to
avoid them. Even the birthday parties and family occasions that
took place in her own home were a torment to her. She repeatedly said that if only she could lose weight she would feel more
confident and then would be much more willing and able to
socialise. The only problem with that argument was that some
years previously she had lost a lot of weight and still she didn't
enjoy socialising. The fact was that she was a very unconfident
person who felt she had nothing to offer at social occasions.
Even though she was a capable woman doing a responsible job
she still felt worthless. The work she needed to do on herself
was to try and improve her self-esteem, not worry about her
weight. As she slowly learned to like and value herself more and
to recognise what she could do and what qualities she had, the
emphasis on her weight shifted; it became less of an issue and she
became much freer to think about whether losing weight was
important to her or whether she could accept herself the way she
was.

3   One of the things we rarely talk about is our own image of

what it means to be a woman. It's probably easier to know
what we don't want to be as women (a drudge, a victim, a sec-
ond-class citizen . . .) One of the problems for many women
about the images offered to us by the media, is that those
skinny, girlish figures are presented as having no value except
as clothes horses or sexual objects. Not many of us are content
with that as a way to think about ourselves. That may be part
of the reason why so few of us actually make ourselves the
shape of models: in more senses than one we feel there is more
to us than that!

Try and make a list of words to describe the kind of woman you
want to be. This is a good exercise to do in a group all together.
When I've done this with groups of clients we've made lists like
this:

strong	brave	laid-back	energetic
funny	caring	unflurried	determined
sexy	creative	calm	fair-minded

Have a go and make your own list.

THE DIFFICULTIES OF GROWING UP

1 One of the very important issues for all of us is the development of our sexuality. How did we develop a sense of
ourselves as women and what are our attitudes towards our
own sexuality? One way of beginning to think about this is to
try and remember what and how you were told about menstruation and by whom. Can you remember the situation?
Sometimes girls are told by other children in a way that is
frightening or puzzling. Probably most girls are told something by their mothers, though what and how varies
enormously. One woman told me her mother had taken her
into her bedroom and sat her down on the bed and then had

closed the curtains, even though it was the middle of the day, before she had started to talk about this very secret matter. How do you think your experience affected you? Can you remember your first menstruation and how you felt about it? Have you a memory of whether you told your mother and how she reacted? Did you cope on your own and if so, what did that feel like?

2 The exercise above can easily be developed further by thinking about how you got to know about sexual intercourse, contraception, pregnancy, delivery and so on. What you were told is probably less important than how you were told – or what you weren't told or didn't know. Try and get in touch with the feelings you had then and consider how that experience has affected you. Many eating disorders seem to be connected with women's difficulties with their sexuality and their relationships with men; try and think whether this might be so for you, and what part your introduction to these subjects has to do with it. For instance, what underlying messages do you think you got about sex? Did you get the idea that it was pleasurable and an ordinary part of adult life, or dirty and to be avoided, or frightening and something that would hurt you? What was implied about men's sexuality and how has that affected you?

3 There has been so much emphasis placed on mother–daughter relationships in trying to understand women, that sometimes father–daughter relationships get lost. Yet, for most of us, the relationship with our father is very important in formulating our attitudes and expectations towards men, and therefore of adult sexual partners. The following exercises are designed to help you begin to explore your relationship with your father.

Turn to page 157 where an exercise on painting you and your mother is described. Try the same exercise for you and your father.

4 There are all sorts of images of fatherhood presented to us by
   our culture: for instance God the Father, Father Christmas,
   Old Father Time, The Godfather. The ideas behind these various images of 'father' are very different. Make a list of words
   that you associate to the word 'father'. When I've done this
   with groups we've come up with lists that have a good many
   contradictions in them, for instance:

strong	punishing	teacher	stern
distant	helper	angry	absent
frightening	kind	loving	nasty
concerned	patient	enemy	violent

   Then go on to make from this list, the list of words that apply
   to your father. What does this list tell you about your attitudes
   to men in general? What effect has your father had on your
   current attitudes and expectations towards men? How has your
   choice of a male partner been affected by your childhood per-
   ceptions of your father? Have you chosen someone like him, or
   unlike him?

One woman I worked with made a list of truly awful characteristics: words such as bully, angry, punishing, spanking, not caring,
brutal, hostile, etc. Not surprisingly she turned out to have had a
very violent, frightening father. The result of all this was that she
saw in every man a potential bully and could not make relationships with men. However she had not consciously known that she
had transferred this image of her father on to every man she came
across. When she saw that this was what she did, she began to be
able to ask herself whether it was in fact true that all men were
like her father.

AT LEAST I'LL CONTROL WHAT
I PUT IN MY MOUTH

One of the key words for any woman with an eating disorder is control. Food is used as the battleground on which she is continually fighting for control, losing control, gaining control. But she has chosen the wrong battleground. The real area in which we need to exercise control is in our lives. That is where the woman with an eating disorder feels she has none.

The following exercises (for which you need at least one other person) are designed to let you explore having and not having control in an area other than food. If you are very worried about control it is highly likely that at some time in your life, probably when you were still a child, you have felt too much under somebody else's control. You need to try and find out what that is about and what feelings you have concerning it. Try the exercises: they may make you feel unreasonably scared or anxious; try and stay with those feelings and let memories and pictures and associations come to your mind. You can ask yourself: 'When have I felt like this before?'; 'What does this remind me of?'; 'Who is it that I think of when I feel like this?' Very likely you will get in touch with parts of your emotional experience that still have lots of strong feelings attached to them. This is where the emotional work needs to be done.

1 Hold hands with someone else. Allow yourself to feel as intensely as you can what emotions are aroused in you by that small physical contact. Maybe the feelings will be a mixture of pleasure and anxiety, maybe more of one than the other. What memories are aroused? How old are you in those memories and what are you feeling?

2 Repeat the above exercise by having someone put an arm round your shoulders. Perhaps this arouses in you a longing to

be cuddled and babied; perhaps it arouses fear and a desire to remove the other person's arm. These two different feelings represent the extremes of a continuum on which we plot ourselves in relation to what we long for and can expect from other people:

total		total
dependence	————————————————	separation
on others		from others

Where do you place yourself on this continuum? Where would you like to be? What are the experiences which have led you to place yourself in the position you choose?

3 Sit on the floor opposite another person, holding both hands. You are going to play a rocking game that you probably played as a child. If you have some music that you can rock to, so much the better. Rock backwards and forwards, allowing yourself to be supported by the other person's weight. Can you allow yourself to trust the other person with your weight? Try and allow yourself to have the emotional experience of alternately supporting and being supported. Which is easier for you? Why do you think that is? What feelings are brought up for you by whichever is more difficult? What do you think that means in terms of your past experience?

4 This is an exercise which is done in a group. Form a tight circle, linking arms. One member of the group should stand in the middle of this small, tight circle. She then holds herself straight and stiff and keeps her feet in one place. Then the group gently pushes her backwards and forwards, using the circle as a container to gently bump her to and fro. Gradually make the circle bigger so that the person in the middle falls further. Obviously the bigger the circle the more trust it takes for

the person in the middle to let herself fall against the ring of people.

Some people do this exercise by not letting themselves feel anything, and others are too frightened to do it at all. If you can, and if you think this exercise could be valuable for you, try it and let it bring up feelings in you.

5 This exercise is the same kind of physical trust exercise as the last one, but is easier to organise if you haven't got a group you can call on. One person should either close her eyes or allow herself to be blindfolded. Her partner then takes her by the arm and leads her about. After a while change places. You can make it more difficult by turning the 'blind' person round several times, so that she loses her sense of direction.

There are very often strong feelings brought up by this exercise, often in both members of the pair. Leading someone else and having responsibility and control can bring up as much anxiety as being the one who is led. In this exercise it is interesting to take note of your fantasies about how the other person will behave, before the exercise has even begun. You may be able to gain some insight into what you expect of other people who have control over you.

6 If you are anxious about control it is highly likely that you exercise control over your breathing, even if you don't do it consciously. Sit very quietly and observe your breathing. How far down does your breath go? What parts of your body move when you breathe? Do you allow the muscles of your abdomen and ribs to help you breathe in or do you only use your chest muscles, so you are sipping the air? Can you breathe out? Try it by seeing how long you can say 'Aaaah' or how long you can sing a note. Try doing this with someone else so that you have

some help to understand what you do when you breathe. It's very difficult to feel anything if you are hardly breathing (which is why we stop breathing when we get a fright) and if you want to be able to deal with your feelings you will have to breathe to discover what they are!

7   Muscle tension is another way in which we try to prevent ourselves from feeling, and control what goes on with us. Think about how your body stores feelings, for instance with headaches, raised shoulders, backache, constipation, muscle cramps, etc. If those uncomfortable parts of you could speak, what would they say? What complaint or sadness or discontent would they have? Try having a conversation with that part of you and see what it says. Once I had a client who couldn't control her bladder very well. She had a conversation that went like this:

Client: Why can I never rely on you? Why are you always leaking and embarrassing me? There's no reason for it, you aren't ill or anything. What's wrong with you for goodness sake?

Bladder: You're so hard on me and so nasty to me. You store everything up and expect me to be able to hold on to it and I can't.

Client: Don't be ridiculous. You don't have to hold any more than any other bladder.

Bladder: I'm not talking about wee, you idiot. I'm talking about all the other things you make me hold. You're so angry and you never let it out. You're never satisfied with yourself and always pushing and striving. I can't stand all the tension and anxiety. It's too much for me.

Client: I didn't know this. You never told me. Am I really like that?

Bladder: I am telling you. That's exactly what I am doing. The trouble is that you haven't been willing to listen.

The point is of course that our bodies know exactly what is going on with us and register all of our experiences and all of our feelings. If we don't listen, or ignore what it's trying to tell us, or use tension or shallow breathing to blot out those messages, then we lose contact with our inner world and our true selves.

MOTHERS AND DAUGHTERS

Unless we try very hard, we are highly likely as females to grow into the women our mothers were. You may be aware of this in some ways: perhaps you find yourself cooking or cleaning in exactly the way your mother did it, whether or not you consciously intend to. Women frequently say that they find themselves using the same phrases and sentences as their mothers did when they speak to their own children, even if those very expressions were intensely irritating to them when they were children themselves. It is very important that we think about and become clearer about the relationship between ourselves and our mothers so that we can make more conscious choices about our own way of being and our own lives. This is often the work of years, but the following exercises are designed to help you make a start on that project, if that seems relevant and appropriate to you.

1   This exercise is another that is probably too hard to do alone. It's ideal for a group to do together. Make a drawing or a painting of your mother and yourself in a background or setting. Spend some time on it – at least 15 minutes if you can – and include as much colour and detail as you can. Remember this is not a test of whether you can paint or not; it is a way of locating unconscious knowledge and feelings about your mother.

When you have finished the painting you can start to think about

what it tells you about your view of the relationship between you
and your mother. If you are in a group, I suggest you each think
about the following points in relation to your own painting and
the paintings of others in the group. Try putting all the paintings
up on the wall, or laying them out on the floor where they can all
be seen at the same time. The differences between the paintings
will stimulate your thinking.

Consider first of all where you have placed the two figures in
relation to the piece of paper. Who is in the centre and who is on
the edge (or nearest to those positions)? Who is higher on the
page and who is lower? If the piece of paper represents your life
space, what does the placing tell you about the importance of
your mother? Second, think about the relative size of the figures
(leaving out for the moment considerations of age)? Does the size
of the child figure tell you anything about how old you see yourself as being in relation to your mother, even now? Then, what
about relative closeness or distance of the figures from each other?
What does that reflect about your closeness to your mother emotionally? Your painting may show you as a child, but the very
fact you chose to paint yourself at that age is important. How old
are you in the picture, and why do you think you painted yourself
at that age? What was the relationship between you and your
mother like at that age? Is there any parallel with the way it is
now?

Then turn to the setting in which you have painted the picture.
Why do you think you chose that setting? If you let your imagi-
nation go free, what does it make you think of to remember that
setting, and what does it make you feel? Then look at the colours
you have chosen. Try and associate with the colours – what do
you think of when you think of blue, for example – and look to
see if you have used the same colours for yourself and your
mother, or different. Then try and use that information to help
you think more about your feelings towards your mother and
yourself. In one group where I used a similar exercise, one

woman's association with the colour of the dress she had painted herself wearing was that it was a 'pretty' colour. That sounds rather pale and uninteresting as an association until she explained that for her to be pretty was what her mother valued most about her. She had to be 'pretty', not dirty or sweaty or crying. That demand from her mother had really shaped her whole life.

These are fairly simple ways of thinking about your picture, but they may help you make a beginning and you may be able to use them as the basis for further thoughts and feelings.

2 Our mothers influence us enormously by what they say as well as by what they do. Make a list of as many typical sayings of your mother as you can remember, for instance: 'I told you so'; 'you should have known better'; 'don't put it down, put it away'; 'I don't like to see that expression on your face'; 'don't answer me back'; etc.

What do you think these phrases and expressions tell you about your mother's view of the world, what was important to her and her attitude to you? I worked with one woman, for instance, who at a conscious level thought of her mother as a sweet, kind generous woman who always thought the best of everyone. She couldn't understand why she and her mother had had such a difficult relationship. Then, when we did this exercise it emerged that her mother's favourite phrases were things like: 'I won't have you saying things like that'; 'if you can't say anything nice don't say anything at all'; 'stop complaining, you're a very lucky girl and don't you forget it'; 'you don't know how lucky you are': etc. So it was true that her mother thought well of everyone, but she also absolutely refused to let her daughter have any complaints or dissatisfactions or disappointments about anyone or anything. Not surprisingly the daughter was seething with all kinds of unexpressed feelings, not least towards her mother.

3   Another avenue to discover the effect your mother has had on
    your identity as a woman, and one that is especially relevant
    for women with eating disorders, is to try and remember what
    your mother's attitude was to her own body and appearance.
    Women who were young in the sixties were the first generation
    to be strongly affected by the cultural pressures for women to
    be thin (Twiggy and all that). If you are the child of a woman
    influenced in that way it is highly likely that your mother was
    anxious or uncertain about her size and shape. Many mothers
    pass on these anxieties to their daughters, so, for example, it is
    not at all unusual for mothers to make their pre-pubescent
    daughters precociously aware of their size and to put them on
    diets, thus starting them on a career of self-consciousness and
    dissatisfaction with their bodies before they are even out of
    childhood. So then, think about your mother's attitude to her
    body. Did she give you an idea of the female body as attractive
    and deserving care and nurture? (And you could think about
    your father's attitude to your mother's body and appearance in
    relation to this.) How carefully did she look after herself in
    relation to things like clothes and hair and make-up and jew-
    ellery? How did she teach you about these things – or at least,
    what do you think you learned from her? Can you see any con-
    nections to your present attitudes and behaviour? One woman
    I worked with was obsessed by the size of her thighs (which
    were as far as I could see, in every way unremarkable). It
    turned out that from the age of 13 she had been nagged by her
    mother on that subject and had gone on endless 'spot-reduc-
    ing' diets, special courses of massage, special exercise regimes
    and so on. It is very difficult to have an uncomplicated attitude
    to your body in the face of that kind of influence.

Where to look next

Ultimately, the decision is your own; you must do what helps you to grow. And you must trust that you are wise enough to know what that is.

Geneen Roth, *Feeding the Hungry Heart*

BOOKS

In this chapter I have gathered together some information which may help you to follow up on the points made and issues raised in this book. I would like to begin with a list of books which I think are useful. They are organised in order of the chapters to which they relate most closely in the book.

Chapter 1
There are several accounts of people who have suffered from eating disorders.

Catherine: a tragic life, Maureen Dunbar (Penguin, 1987).
Catherine was a young woman who died of anorexia. This book is written by Catherine's mother with sections by her father and brother. It is a sad, but also a very disturbing story of how no appropriate or effective treatment could be found for Catherine and how her behaviour patterns hardened until no intervention of any kind was possible. In terms of this book it is particularly interesting because it shows how food was an available metaphor in the family for Catherine to use; from the very beginning she

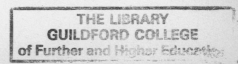

had had difficulties with food and eating which were allowed to become a source of conflict. It is also the story of a family in which there were all sorts of emotional disturbances and turmoil which deeply affected Catherine. Her own account of why she stopped eating in the first place was that she was trying to have an effect on the family situation. Most of all it is a book which demonstrates that responding to an eating disorder as if it were about food does not work.

The Art of Starvation, Sheila Macleod (Virago, 1981).
This is an autobiographical account of a period of anorexia, 20 years previously, by a woman who is a writer. It is particularly interesting in that she discusses her experience in relation to the various theories about anorexia and tries to show where they fit with her experience and where they don't. Like the account of Catherine, it is the story of someone who at the time got no psychological help, although Macleod's illness was much less severe and never became chronic.

Dancing on my Grave, Gelsey Kirkland (Hamish Hamilton, 1987).
Gelsey Kirkland was an American ballet dancer, 'one of the most dazzling ballerinas of her generation', who danced with Mikhail Baryshnikov and as a star of Balanchine's company, New York City Ballet. Her career was brought to a brutal and untimely end by her serious emotional illnesses which resulted in anorexia and drug addiction. This is a very shocking book, not least because it describes the hostility and indifference of the dance world to the emotional pain of a phenomenally gifted dancer. Gelsey Kirkland talks very openly about her life, without, I think, having much understanding of how it came to be that way, and what part she played in allowing and making it that way.

Elizabeth Takes Off, Elizabeth Taylor (Pan, 1988).
A curiously honest, moving and dignified book which tells Elizabeth Taylor's life story in terms of the relationship between

her emotional life and her weight gains and losses. The second half of the book is a more or less standard diet book, but with quite a lot of interesting comment and advice about the psychological strain of losing weight.

The Fat Woman's Joke, Fay Weldon (Coronet, 1982).
This is a quite extraordinary novel which describes how a married couple dealt with the conflict and difficulties of their marriage by a shared pattern of compulsive eating. The preoccupation with food takes the socially condoned form of gourmet eating. When they both decide to go on a diet the violence and hostility that lurks below the surface immediately becomes apparent. The woman leaves and immediately tries to heal the agonising void that has become apparent with frantic, uncontrolled, compulsive eating; the man uses sex for the same purpose. A painful story.

Feeding the Hungry Heart, Geneen Roth (Signet, 1982).
Although Roth starts from the same premise as this book, that compulsive eating seeks to express some unhappiness, her chief concern is to describe the experience of being a compulsive eater. She has assembled a book of pieces of writing describing how an emotional trigger finally goads a compulsive eater into a binge. There are many beautifully written and moving accounts of terrible moments in people's lives, most of them written by participants in Roth's workshops. Through it all she stresses the overwhelming need for us to accept and love ourselves more.

Lifesize, Jenefer Shute, (Secker and Warburg, 1992).
This is a novel describing the experience of an anorexic in hospital who is trying to learn to eat again. A vivid and touching account.

Chapter 2
The Child, the Family and the Outside World, D.W. Winnicott (Pelican, 1973).
D.W. Winnicott was a distinguished psychiatrist and analyst who

spent many years working with mothers and small children. He had the gift of expressing his ideas in a way that was both charming and accessible. In the 1950s he gave some talks on the radio which eventually became the basis of this book. Some of it is now a little dated, but it is also, I think, an amazingly tender and wise book. It is particularly touching on the feeding relationship of mother and child.

Chapter 4
Fat is a Feminist Issue, Susie Orbach (Arrow Books, 1988).
By far the most interesting and exciting writing about understanding eating disorders has been done by feminist writers in the last 15 years. It will be clear from what I have said earlier in the book that I don't consider a feminist understanding to be the *only* way of thinking about eating disorders, but it is certainly a very valuable way.

The most distinguished book is that by Susie Orbach. Its value can be seen by its publication history. It has been repeatedly reprinted since the first edition in 1978 and the edition given here is merely the latest in a long line. The basic thesis of the book is that 'compulsive eating in women is a response to their social position'.

Hunger Strike: the anorexic's struggle as a metaphor for our age, Susie Orbach (Faber and Faber, 1987).
Fat is a Feminist Issue has been followed up by Orbach with a book on anorexia. In this quite difficult book Orbach presents anorexia as an exaggerated and extravagant response to the cultural demand that women should be thin, small, invisible. The anorexic overperforms and in so doing not only shows her own pain but the violence of the sociological pressures acting on her.

Women's Secret Disorder: A new understanding of Bulimia, Mira Dana and Marilyn Lawrence (Grafton Books, 1988).

This is a book which tries to understand bulimia from a feminist perspective. In places it is quite a difficult book, but with a great deal of very valuable material in it, particularly since so little has been written on bulimia.

Fed Up and Hungry: Women, Oppression and Food, Marilyn Lawrence (ed.) (Women's Press, 1987).
A valuable and interesting collection of papers from a feminist perspective about eating disorders in women.

Womansize, Kim Chernin (Women's Press, 1983).
This book explores the idea that women are required to be thin because our culture hates and fears women and women's bodies. Chernin talks about men's envy of women's power to conceive, bear and suckle children and of the power of a woman's body for all of us when we were infants. Because women also have mixed memories of our infant experience of the power of a woman's body, we are also afraid of the size and power of our own bodies. For this reason we agree to follow the cultural demand that our bodies become weak, small and powerless.

Chapter 5
There aren't enough books that discuss the difficult transition from child to adult via adolescence but you may be able to find useful sections in these two.

Families and How to Survive Them, Robin Skynner and John Cleese (Methuen, 1983). Ten years on from publication I think it's still the best book to help you begin to understand what was going on in your family and how to recognise how that has affected you.

Secrets in the Family, Lily Pincus and Christopher Dare (Faber and Faber, 1978).

Chapter 6
The Golden Cage: the enigma of anorexia nervosa, Hilde Bruch
(Open Books, 1978).
Hilde Bruch was a distinguished pioneer in the better understanding of anorexia when it was still known as an illness of
prosperous middle-class, over-protective families. It was she who
described the necessity of children and youngsters having space
and opportunity to make their own decisions and identify their
own needs and wants. She saw anorexics as young women determined to create an area of control in their own lives.

She draws attention to the long preparation that goes on setting
the scene for anorexia in this kind of family, especially the anorexic's
feeling that she has to be what her parents want her to be and the
consequent need always to be guessing and figuring out what that
might be. Bruch suggests that the anorexic lacks the ability to be a
normally selfish and self-absorbed child, so that she is consumed
with anxiety about what 'other people' think of her. Assertiveness,
anger, protest and discontent are all completely unknown.

Bruch also points out what an unmanageable struggle puberty
and adolescence pose to such young women, because of changes
that they cannot accept in their bodies and minds, and because of
the self-assertion that adolescence demands. They are stuck devel-
opmentally as children.

Chapter 7
Our Mothers' Daughters, Judith Arcana (Womens Press, 1981).
A sympathetic account of the relationship between mothers and
daughters.

The Hungry Self, Kim Chernin (Virago, 1986).
This book explores the connection between mother–daughter
relationships and eating disorders. Chernin is particularly interested in the issue of separation and the way in which daughters
are so much in touch with their mother's pain.

Chapter 8
The Courage to Heal: A Guide for Women Survivors of Child Sexual Abuse, Ellen Bass and Laura Davis (Harper and Row, 1988).
An absolutely first rate book. Highly recommended.

Chapter 9
Understanding Women, Susie Orbach and Luise Eichenbaum (Penguin, 1985).
This quite remarkable book is a major contribution to the under-· standing of women's emotional development. Much thinking on emotional development has either concentrated on male emotional development or has assumed that male and female development were the same. In the past several decades all sorts of studies have made it very obvious that from the very beginning boy and girl babies are treated differently. This book gives a fascinating analysis of the particular pressures and expectations for girls as they grow up and provides the theoretical underpinning for Orbach's other books.

Our Need for Others and its Roots in infancy, Josephine Klein (Tavistock, 1987).
A lovely book. Readers should not be put off by a couple of very technical and scientific chapters early in the book. This book provides a very interesting account of human emotional development which could very well be read alongside Orbach and Eichenbaum.

When Food is Love, Geneen Roth (Piatkus,1991).
The latest from G.R. and in my view the best. She addresses the problems of learning how to relate when your childhood experience hasn't taught you to do it well.

Toxic Parents, Susan Forward (Bantam, 1989).
An excellent and very readable self-help book for those from disturbed and distressed backgrounds.

Chapter 10
There are several books which contribute to the practical response to an eating disorder.

Two of these are by Paulette Maisner, herself a former sufferer from eating disorders, and founder of the Maisner Centre, 57a Church Road, Hove, East Sussex BN3 2BD. Telephone: (0273) 729818/29334.

The Food Trap: a self-help plan to control your eating habits, Paulette Maisner with Rosemary Turner (Unwin Paperbacks, 1986).

Excuses Won't Cure You, Paulette Maisner with Alison Cridland (Unwin, 1987).
Maisner is concerned with a different aspect of eating disorders from the one that has been explored in this book. Her books are intended to educate the reader in how to eat properly, what different food values are, how to exercise beneficially, how to deal with practical aspects of breaking the habit of food misuse. She is clear that this is her field of expertise and not the underlying emotional problems. Her response to these is very commonsensical and bracing.

Fat is a Feminist Issue 2, Susie Orbach (Hamlyn, 1984).
This is the practical follow-up and accompaniment to *Fat is a Feminist Issue*. The ideas that it is based on are the feminist understanding of compulsive eating of her earlier book, so it has special interest to readers of this book who have found Chapter Four particularly relevant to them. However, because Orbach starts from the same assumption as this book, that eating disorders are not just about eating, the strategies and exercises she suggests are very much in line with much of what has been said here. One of the most interesting sections is on how to set up a compulsive eating group and thus create a support network for yourself.

Breaking Free from Compulsive Eating, Geneen Roth (Grafton Books, 1986).
A lovely book, full of exercises to get in touch with what your wants and needs are. Also a lot of ideas on how to become more conscious of how, what, where and when you eat. There is also a lot to help towards self-acceptance.

Coping with Bulimia, Barbara French (Grafton, 1987).
An encouraging and helpful book with a lot of useful information and a gentle supportive style.

In Our Own Hands, Sheila Ernst and Lucy Goodison (Women's Press, 1981).
This is a self-help book for women who want to think about themselves and their emotional development. A wonderful book, useful, interesting, practical and full of good ideas.

The Anorexia Nervosa Reference Book, Roger Slade (Harper and Row, 1984).
A question and answer book with a lot of information.

The Courage to Heal: A Guide for Women Survivors of Child Sexual Abuse, Ellen Bass and Laura Davis (Harper and Row, 1988).
If you want to work on your experience of sexual abuse, the best advice I can give you is to get hold of this book.

Families and How to Survive Them, Robin Skynner and John Cleese (Methuen, 1983).
When people come to me bothered about their relationships, I often suggest that they read this book together as a way of discovering what their families of origin were like. Valuable reading.

Toxic Parents, Susan Forward (Bantam, 1989).
I recommend this book to those who have the sort of dreadful family background described in Chapter 10.

MEDICAL HELP

One of the awful things about eating disorders is that they can do terrible damage to our bodies. Food misusers complain of a very wide range of physical symptoms which can be traced back to their eating behaviour. There are also a number of quite rare conditions that mimic the symptoms of an eating disorder and it is desirable to eliminate that possibility. Mostly, food misusers are so ashamed of their difficulties that they find it very difficult to be honest with a doctor and will usually provide him or her with only part of the information necessary to understand what is going on. Understandably the response is then not usually very helpful. It is also true that some doctors have no clue about the emotional anguish of a food misuser and can be impatient or dismissive. On the other hand, there are also patient and concerned GPs who will offer support and carry out blood tests and so on which can identify (for example) mineral imbalance as a result of bulimia, hormonal disturbances in the compulsive eater, or deficiency states as a result of anorexia.

Doctors also often have basic nutritional information and sample menus which can be helpful to the food misuser who has lost all sense of how much is a good amount to eat or of what. In fact it has been my experience that food misusers often just do not know what their bodies need or what an ordinary diet looks like. Sometimes such people come from households where eating behaviour was chaotic. Others may have been brought up in institutions where food was provided at certain times and in certain quantities. Sometimes normal eating patterns have been disrupted for so long that a sense of how ordinary people eat has been lost. When such people have to sort out for themselves what to eat, how much and when, they can feel utterly overwhelmed.

Doctors in Britain are also the route to NHS psychological help. If you want that kind of help then you will almost certainly have to begin with your GP. If you don't like or don't trust your

GP, then find another. You have no obligation to go on seeing the GP with whom you are registered. If you attend college there will certainly be a doctor attached to the College Health Service. That doctor is also very likely to be familiar with eating disorders. If you hear of a GP that you think you would prefer to your own you can ask to transfer if you live within the geographical area covered by that practice. Sometimes women prefer to see women doctors. You can ask to see a woman in a group practice where there are both men and women.

HELPING YOURSELF PSYCHOLOGICALLY

The material in this book has mostly come from my experience as a counsellor working with people who are bothered about the way they use food. Some people may want to look for counselling or other professional help to carry further what they have learned about themselves through using this book. I will try to outline the kind of help that is available. However, I would first like to describe how to go about helping yourself further if you don't want professional help.

Obviously you can read more. Susie Orbach's *Hunger Strike* has a section which is especially addressed to anorexics who want to try and work on themselves. All of the books listed above are worth looking at. However, for most of us other human beings are what we need. Support groups are often helpful. *Fat is a Feminist Issue 2* describes in detail how to set one up, as do Goodison and Ernst in *In Our Own Hands* and Dana and Lawrence in *Women's Secret Disorder*. There is an organisation for anorexics and bulimics which offers support and information:

The Eating Disorders Association
This organisation offers help and understanding around anorexia and bulimia, and incorporates Anorexic Aid and Anorexic Family

Aid, which have both been going for some time. For further details contact:

The Eating Disorders Association
Sackville Place
44 Magdalen Street
Norwich
Norfolk NR3 1JE
Telephone: 0603 621414

There is also an organisation called **Overeaters Anonymous** (OA) which works on the same lines as Alcoholics Anonymous, with mutual support from recovering fellow-sufferers. Their contact address is:

140a Tachbrook Street
London SW1
Telephone: 071-834 8202

Their literature is available from Quest Books, River House, 46 Lea Road, Waltham Abbey, Essex EN9 1AT.

The Women's Therapy Centre
6–9 Manor Gardens
London N7
Telephone: 071-263 6200

This organisation runs two-day courses for women thinking of setting up self-help eating disorder support groups.

Often those who start work on themselves after a while think they might like also to use some professional help.

PSYCHOLOGICAL HELP FROM PROFESSIONALS

The National Health Service

The first contact should be with your GP. Some GPs are interested in and informed about psychological issues and will be willing to offer you counselling themselves. Pressures on a GP's time, however, are very likely to make this help quite short term and you will probably not be given sessions longer than half an hour. However, that may be long enough, or at least enough to be going on with. On the other hand, many GPs don't do that kind of psychological work and will want to refer you on.

The first possibility may be a counsellor who belongs to the medical practice. Increasingly group practices and health centres are employing counsellors. Again these services are under pressure and you are likely to be offered a limited number of sessions. However, these will be with someone who is trained to deal with psychological issues.

If the practice does not have a counsellor then the next port of call by this route is the outpatient department of a psychiatric hospital or a department of psychological medicine. These vary enormously in their competence to deal with psychological issues. Psychiatrists are doctors who have had a further training in psychiatry. That training has been very largely in the administration of drugs to people who are mentally ill. However, it is increasingly possible for psychiatrists to do psychotherapy training which educates them in psychological issues, and some do. There are also clinical psychologists working in hospitals who are not concerned with the administration of drugs, but with psychology. In addition to that, some hospitals have units that are specifically concerned with food misuse, usually anorexia and bulimia. Some hospitals have family therapy departments which can be useful for younger people still living at home. There are also adolescent units attached to some hospitals.

All of these services are over-stretched and you are likely to have to wait several weeks at least for an initial appointment unless you are seriously ill as a result of your eating disorder. The entire psychiatric hospital service is primarily geared towards seriously ill people and to their treatment with drugs. You need psychotherapy rather than this sort of treatment, and it is a matter of trying to locate that within the system. Your GP should be able to help.

This does not quite exhaust the provision of counselling and psychotherapy within the NHS. There are some clinics set up explicitly to deal with psychological problems, but not within psychiatric hospitals or departments. In Oxford there is the ISIS Centre which is the only self-referral counselling centre in the country under the NHS. It is specifically set up for people who are not mentally ill, but who are troubled about some aspect of their lives. In London there is the Tavistock Clinic and the Paddington Centre. These both offer psychotherapy within a restricted catchment area via GP referral. All of these offer excellent therapy within a reasonable time-span, although you will be put on a waiting list. There may well be other such clinics elsewhere. Your GP should know of them.

OTHER AGENCIES

If none of the above seems very hopeful, there are some alternatives, some free some with means tested fees and some entirely private.

If you are under 16 there is a system of Child and Family Clinics. Some of these are very good indeed and you can refer yourself. They are part of the social services provision and cost nothing to the users. Although some are behavioural in their orientation, some offer psychotherapy and family therapy.

If you are a student in further education or higher education, it is very likely that your institution will have a counsellor. At the very least your **college health service** will be able to refer you.

There is a whole range of counselling agencies. Some of these are highly specific – such as Rape Crisis – but some offer much more general counselling. Three books that may help you find your way round the counselling world are *Talking to a Stranger* by L. Knight (Fontana, 1986), *Counselling Shop* by Brigid Proctor (Burnett Books, 1978) and *Individual Therapy in Britain* edited by Windy Dryden (Harper Row, 1984). It is very important that you find the kind of counselling and a counsellor that suits you. If you don't feel comfortable or happy with your first choice, try again.

Two nationwide agencies that both do excellent work are the **Samaritans** and **Relate** (formerly the Marriage Guidance Council). Both of these have developed their work considerably and are no longer solely concerned with the specific problems they were originally established to respond to. Relate asks for a contribution to the cost of its counselling sessions. The Samaritans offers free counselling, especially for crisis and emergency. Their local numbers are in the telephone directory.

The British Association for Counselling (BAC), 1 Regent Place, Rugby CV21 3BX, is the professional association for counsellors and publishes a *Counselling and Psychotherapy Resources Directory*. This is a useful guide by area, although it is not exhaustive. Public libraries and town halls may also have details of local counselling agencies. Many counselling agencies (as opposed to individual counsellors) are supported by public or charitable money and consequently either do not charge, charge nominal sums or charge according to a means tested scale.

The work done by counselling agencies is usually short term and problem-solving in its approach. A more long term approach is offered by psychotherapy. Since May 1993 psychotherapists in Britain who have trained with an approved organisation and are regarded as competent to practise have been included on a National Register of Psychotherapists. This can be consulted by phoning 071-487 7554. Here are some organisations which you can approach:

The Womens Therapy Centre, 6 Manor Gardens, London N7, has a referral service for individual psychotherapy and also runs workshops and groups for women with eating disorders.

The British Association of Psychotherapists runs a clinic offering low-cost therapy.
37 Mapesbury Rd
London NW2 4HJ
Telephone: 081-452 9823

The Guild of Psychotherapists offers a country-wide referral service.
19b Thornton Hill
London SW19 4HU

People with eating disorders nearly always have serious difficulties in liking the way they look. Interest is growing in how Dance Movement Therapy can help with these difficulties. To contact dance movement therapists write to:
The Association for Dance Movement Therapy
c/o The Arts Therapies Dept
Springfield Hospital
61 Glenburnie Rd
London SW17 7DJ

The author of this book continues with a private practice and also lectures and runs seminars and workshops on eating disorders. She can be contacted at the following address:
Julia Buckroyd
Principle Lecturer in Counselling
University of Hertfordshire
Meridian House
Common Road
Hertford, Herts, AL10 0NZ

Index